# Contents

# Contributors

**Susan E. Antczak,** RN, OCN
*Clinical Instructor, CNA/MA Program*
Fox Chase Cancer Center
Philadelphia

**Nancy Berger,** RN, BC, MSN
*Instructor*
Charles E. Gregory School of Nursing
Raritan Bay Medical Center
Perth Amboy, N.J.

**Wendy Tagan Conroy,** RN, MSN, FNP, BC
*Advanced Practice Registered Nurse*
Saint Francis Hospital and Medical Center
Hartford, Conn.

**Lillian Craig,** RN, CS, FNP
*Family Nurse Practitioner*
Claude Rural Health Clinic
Claude, Tex.

**Shelba Durston,** RN, MSN, CCRN
*Staff Nurse*
San Joaquin General Hospital
French Camp, Calif.
*Faculty*
San Joaquin Delta College
Stockton, Calif.

**Deborah A. Hanes,** RN, MSN, CNS, NPC
*Clinical Nurse Specialist – Cardiovascular Surgery/ Stepdown*
The Cleveland Clinic Foundation
Cleveland

**Joyce Lyne Heise,** RN, MSN, EdD
*Associate Professor of Nursing*
Kent State University
East Liverpool, Ohio

**Carol T. Lemay,** RN
*Staff Observation/Triage Nurse*
University of Massachusetts
Amherst

**Concha Carillo Sitter,** RN, MS,
   APN, CGRN, FNP
*GI Nurse Practitioner*
Sterling Rock Falls Clinic
Sterling, Ill.

**Robin R. Wilkerson,** RN, PhD,
   BC
*Associate Professor*
University of Mississippi School
   of Nursing
Jackson, Miss.

# Foreword

Every experienced nurse or clinician knows that understanding the underlying mechanisms and pathologic effects of disease is key to providing quality, individualized, up-to-the-minute care. And, as every student or recent graduate soon discovers, gleaning such essential information from various textbooks, journals, and other references to form a solid nursing knowledge base can be a daunting, highly complex undertaking.

*Just the Facts: Pathophysiology* is an excellent resource for both students and seasoned nurses alike—anyone who needs a clear, concise review of the underlying mechanisms and physiologic changes that occur with the most commonly encountered diseases and disorders. All of the chapters in this well-organized book follow the same basic format, ensuring quick and easy access to only the most essential information on each disease state.

The book is arranged primarily by body systems (Chapters 1 through 11), followed by individual chapters on genetic disorders (Chapter 12) and disorders of fluids, electrolytes, and acid-base balance (Chapter 13). Each chapter begins with a succinct overview of the major pathophysiologic concepts specific to that body system or overall problem, followed by individual, alphabetized entries covering some of the most common diseases and disorders (a discussion of less common diseases can be found in the Appendix).

Within each entry, readers will find only the most relevant information—just the facts—in the form of bulleted introductory comments, a list of associated causes, a two-column presentation of pathophysiologic changes, and a compilation of the most current nursing and medical management practices. Each chapter also contains numerous graphic illustrations and helpful flowcharts depicting significant mechanisms leading to disease. Recurring icons (*The Patho Picture, Pathophysiologic Changes, How It Happens,* and *Management*) enable readers to quickly locate information and to compare or contrast findings among related disease entries.

Whether used as a quick-reference guide or as an adjunct to more detailed textbooks or clinical courses, *Just the Facts: Pathophysiology* is an indispensable tool that will help practicing nurses and students of all levels to recognize abnormal body changes, understand how diseases develop, and determine appropriate treatment options—all essential to providing exceptional nursing care.

**Joan Tilghman,** RN, PhD
*Assistant Professor, Division of Nursing*
Howard University
Washington, D.C.

# 1

# Cardiovascular disorders

## Pathophysiologic concepts   2

## Disorders   6

# PATHOPHYSIOLOGIC CONCEPTS

## *Aneurysm*

- ◆ Localized outpouching or dilation of weakened arterial wall
- ◆ Can result from atherosclerotic plaque formation, loss of elastin and collagen in vessel wall, congenital abnormalities in media of arterial wall, trauma, infection

---

### TYPES OF AORTIC ANEURYSM

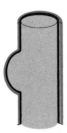

**Saccular aneurysm**
Unilateral pouchlike bulge with narrow neck

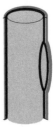

**Dissecting aneurysm**
Hemorrhagic separation of medial layers of vessel wall, which create false lumen

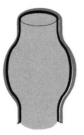

**Fusiform aneurysm**
Spindle-shaped bulge encompassing entire diameter of vessel

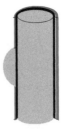

**False aneurysm**
Pulsating hematoma resulting from trauma and commonly mistaken for abdominal aneurysm

**COMMON LOCATIONS**
◆ Abdominal aorta, between renal arteries and iliac branches
◆ Thoracic aorta (ascending, transverse, or descending)
◆ Cerebral artery, at arterial junction in circle of Willis
◆ Femoral and popliteal arteries

## Cardiac shunt

◆ Provides "communication" between pulmonary and systemic circulations
◆ Blood flows from area of high pressure to area of low pressure or from area of high resistance to area of low resistance

**LEFT-TO-RIGHT SHUNT**
◆ Blood flows through atrial or ventricular defect or from aorta to pulmonary circulation through patent ductus arteriosus
◆ Delivers oxygenated blood back to right side of heart or to lungs
◆ If congenital, called an acyanotic defect
◆ Pulmonary blood flow increases as blood is continually recirculated to lungs
◆ Leads to hypertrophy of pulmonary vessels and possible right-sided heart failure

**RIGHT-TO-LEFT SHUNT**
◆ Blood flows from right side of heart to left (such as in tetralogy of Fallot) or from pulmonary artery directly into systemic circulation through patent ductus arteriosus
◆ Adds deoxygenated blood to systemic circulation
◆ Leads to hypoxia and cyanosis
◆ If congenital, called a cyanotic defect
◆ Manifestations: fatigue, increased respiratory rate, clubbing of fingers

## *Embolus*

- ◆ Substance that circulates from one location in body to another through bloodstream
- ◆ Most emboli are blood clots from thrombus
- ◆ May also consist of pieces of tissue, an air bubble, amniotic fluid, fat, bacteria, tumor cells, or foreign substance

### *VENOUS EMBOLI*

- ◆ Originate in venous circulation
- ◆ Travel to right side of heart and pulmonary circulation
- ◆ Eventually lodge in capillary

### *ARTERIAL EMBOLI*

- ◆ Originate in left side of heart from arrhythmias, valvular heart disease, myocardial infarction (MI), heart failure, or endocarditis
- ◆ May lodge in organs (such as brain, kidneys) or extremities

## *Release of cardiac enzymes and proteins*

- ◆ Damaged heart muscle, impaired integrity of cell membrane
- ◆ Triggers release of intracellular cardiac enzymes (creatine kinase, lactate dehydrogenase, and aspartate aminotransferase) and proteins (troponin T, troponin I, and myoglobin) in characteristic rising and falling of cardiac values

## *Stenosis*

- ◆ Narrowing blood vessel or heart valve
- ◆ Tissues and organs perfused by stenosed blood vessel; may become ischemic, function abnormally, or die
- ◆ Blood accumulates in chamber behind stenosed valve; resistance of stenosed valve increases chamber pressure
- ◆ Hypertrophy may result
- ◆ Stenosis of valve on left side of heart increases pulmonary venous pressure and pulmonary congestion, leading to right-sided heart failure
- ◆ Stenosis of valve on right side of heart leads to systemic venous congestion

## *Thrombus*

◆ Blood clot (consisting of platelets, fibrin, and red and white blood cells) that forms anywhere within vascular system
◆ Three conditions (Virchow's triad) that promote thrombus formation
    – Endothelial injury: attracts platelets and other inflammatory mediators, which may stimulate clot formation
    – Sluggish blood flow: allows platelets and clotting factors to accumulate and adhere to blood vessel walls
    – Increased coagulability: promotes clot formation
◆ Consequences: occluded blood vessel, embolus

## *Valve incompetence*

◆ Occurs when valve leaflets don't completely close
◆ May affect valves of veins or heart
◆ When vein valve leaflets close improperly, blood flows backward and pools above, causing valve to weaken and become incompetent
◆ Veins eventually become distended, resulting in varicose veins, chronic venous insufficiency, and venous stasis ulcers
◆ Blood clots may form as blood flow becomes sluggish
◆ Incompetent heart valves allow blood to flow in both directions through valve
◆ Volume of blood pumped increases
◆ Involved heart chambers dilate to accommodate increased volume

# DISORDERS

## Acute coronary syndrome

◆ Begins with rupture or erosion of plaque
◆ Results in platelet adhesions, fibrin clot formation, and activation of thrombin
◆ Degree of coronary artery occlusion determines whether ACS is unstable angina, non–Q-wave MI, or Q-wave MI

**THE PATHO PICTURE**

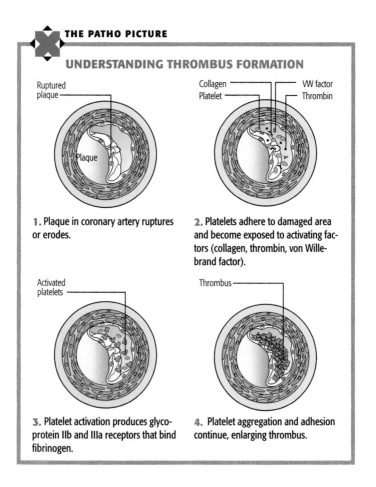

### UNDERSTANDING THROMBUS FORMATION

**1.** Plaque in coronary artery ruptures or erodes.

**2.** Platelets adhere to damaged area and become exposed to activating factors (collagen, thrombin, von Willebrand factor).

**3.** Platelet activation produces glycoprotein IIb and IIIa receptors that bind fibrinogen.

**4.** Platelet aggregation and adhesion continue, enlarging thrombus.

## *Causes*

- ◆ Atherosclerosis
- ◆ Embolism

## *Risk factors*

- ◆ Family history of heart disease
- ◆ Obesity, sedentary lifestyle
- ◆ Smoking
- ◆ High-fat, high-carbohydrate diet
- ◆ Menopause
- ◆ Stress
- ◆ Diabetes
- ◆ Hypertension
- ◆ Hyperlipoproteinemia

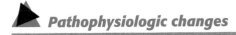 *Pathophysiologic changes*

### IN ANGINA

Myocardial ischemia ➡ Chest pain (burning, squeezing, or crushing)
– Usually in substernal or precordial chest
– May radiate to left arm, neck, jaw, or shoulder blade
– Relieved by nitroglycerin

### IN MI

Coronary artery occlusion ➡ Chest pain (severe, persistent, crushing, or squeezing)
– Usually in substernal chest
– May radiate to left arm, jaw, neck, or shoulder blade
– Goes unrelieved by rest or nitroglycerin

Pain; sympathetic stimulation ➡ Perspiration; anxiety; hypertension; feeling of impending doom

Impaired myocardial function ➡ Fatigue; shortness of breath; cool extremities; hypotension

Pain; vagal stimulation ➡ Nausea and vomiting

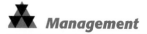 *Management*

### FOR ANGINA

◆ Nitrates — *to reduce myocardial oxygen consumption*
◆ Beta-adrenergic blockers — *to reduce heart's workload and oxygen demands*
◆ Calcium channel blockers — *to treat angina caused by coronary artery spasm*
◆ Antiplatelet drugs — *to minimize platelet aggregation and danger of coronary occlusion*
◆ Antilipemic drugs — *to reduce elevated serum cholesterol or triglyceride levels*
◆ Coronary artery bypass surgery or percutaneous transluminal coronary angioplasty — *for obstructive lesions*

### FOR MI

◆ Thrombolytic therapy (unless contraindicated) within 3 hours of onset of symptoms — *to restore vessel patency and minimize necrosis*
◆ PTCA — *to open blocked or narrowed arteries*
◆ Oxygen — *to increase oxygenation of blood*
◆ Nitroglycerin sublingually — *to relieve chest pain* (unless systolic blood pressure < 90 mm Hg or heart rate < 50 or > 100 beats/minute)
◆ Morphine — *to relieve pain*
◆ Aspirin — *to inhibit platelet aggregation*
◆ I.V. heparin (for patients who have received tissue plasminogen activator) — *to promote patency in affected coronary artery*
◆ Lidocaine, transcutaneous pacing patches (or transvenous pacemaker), defibrillation, or epinephrine — *to combat arrhythmias*
◆ I.V. nitroglycerin for 24 to 48 hours (in patients without hypotension, bradycardia, or excessive tachycardia) — *to reduce afterload and preload and relieve chest pain*
◆ Glycoprotein IIb/IIIa inhibitors (with continued unstable angina or acute chest pain or after invasive cardiac procedures) — *to reduce platelet aggregation*

# Aneurysm, abdominal aortic

◆ Abnormal dilation in aortic arterial wall
◆ Generally occurs between renal arteries and iliac branches

## HOW IT HAPPENS

Degenerative changes occur in aorta.

Focal weakness develops in muscular layer of aorta (tunica media).

Inner layer (tunica intima) and outer layer (tunica adventicia) stretch outward.

Blood pressure within aorta progressively weakens vessel walls.

Aneurysm enlarges.

## *Causes*

◆ Arteriosclerosis
◆ Cystic medial necrosis
◆ Trauma
◆ Syphilis and other infections

## 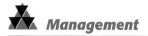 *Pathophysiologic changes*

Enlargement of aorta ➤    Pulsatile mass in periumbilical area

Turbulent blood flow ➤    Systolic bruit over aorta

Pressure on lumbar nerves ➤    Lumbar pain that radiates to flank and groin; severe, persistent abdominal and back pain

Hemorrhage ➤    Weakness, sweating, tachycardia, hypotension

## *Management*

◆ Regular physical examination and ultrasound checks — *to detect enlargement (which may forewarn rupture)*
◆ Risk factor modification, including control of hypocholesterolemia and hypertension — *to prevent expansion and rupture*
◆ Beta blockers — *to reduce risk of aneurysm expansion and rupture*
◆ Resection of aneurysm and replacement of damaged aortic section with Dacron graft — *to repair aneurysm*
◆ Monitoring for signs of acute blood loss (decreasing blood pressure; increasing pulse and respiratory rate; cool, clammy skin; restlessness; decreased sensorium) — *to detect signs of rupture*
◆ Immediate surgery — *to treat rupture* (if needed)

# Aortic insufficiency

◆ Incomplete closure of aortic valve
◆ Usually results from scarring or retraction of valve leaflets

**THE PATHO PICTURE**

**UNDERSTANDING THROMBUS FORMATION**

Blood flows back into the left ventricle during diastole, causing fluid overload in the ventricle, which dilates and hypertrophies. The excess volume causes fluid overload in the left atrium and, finally, the pulmonary system. Left-sided heart failure and pulmonary edema eventually result.

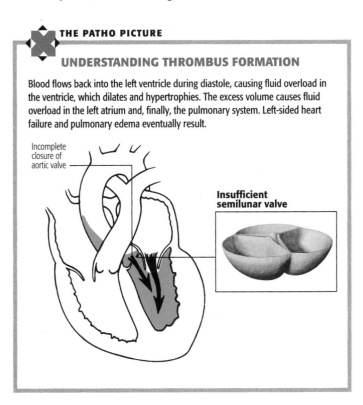

Incomplete closure of aortic valve

**Insufficient semilunar valve**

## *Causes*

### *ACUTE AORTIC INSUFFICIENCY*

- Endocarditis
- Chest trauma
- Prosthetic valve malfunction
- Acute ascending aortic dissection

### *CHRONIC AORTIC INSUFFICIENCY*

- Hypertension
- Rheumatic fever
- Marfan syndrome
- Ankylosing spondylitis
- Syphilis
- Ventricular septal defect

## *Pathophysiologic changes*

### *ACUTE AORTIC INSUFFICIENCY*

| | |
|---|---|
| Left ventricular failure ➡ | Pulmonary congestion and possible cardiogenic shock |

### *CHRONIC AORTIC INSUFFICIENCY*

| | |
|---|---|
| Increased pulmonary venous pressure and cardiac dysfunction ➡ | Exertional dyspnea, orthopnea, and paroxysmal nocturnal dyspnea |
| Left ventricular dysfunction ➡ | Fatigue, exercise intolerance, pulmonary congestion, left-sided heart failure, "pulsating" nail beds (Quincke's sign), $S_3$ heart sound |
| Inadequate coronary perfusion ➡ | Angina |
| Hyperdynamic and tachycardic left ventricle ➡ | Palpitations |
| Low diastolic pressure ➡ | Widened pulse pressure |
| Regurgitant blood flow ➡ | Diastolic blowing murmur at left sternal border |

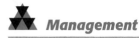 *Management*

### ACUTE AORTIC INSUFFICIENCY

◆ Oxygen — *to increase oxygenation*
◆ Dobutamine — *to reduce afterload*
◆ Vasodilators — *to reduce systolic load and regurgitant volume*
◆ Valve replacement with prosthetic valve — *to remove diseased aortic valve*

### CHRONIC AORTIC INSUFFICIENCY

◆ Vasodilators — *to reduce systolic load and regurgitant volume*
◆ Digoxin, low-sodium diet, diuretic — *to treat left-sided heart failure*
◆ Prophylactic antibiotics before and after surgery or dental care — *to prevent endocarditis*
◆ Nitroglycerin — *to relieve angina*
◆ Valve replacement with prosthetic valve — *to remove diseased aortic valve*

# Aortic stenosis

◆ Narrowing of aortic valve
◆ Classified as acquired or rheumatic
◆ Classic triad of angina pectoris, syncope, and dyspnea

**THE PATHO PICTURE**

### UNDERSTANDING AORTIC STENOSIS

Stenosis of the aortic valve results in impedance to forward blood flow. The left ventricle requires greater pressure to open the aortic valve. The added workload increases the demand for oxygen, and diminished cardiac output causes poor coronary artery perfusion, ischemia of the left ventricle, left ventricular hypertrophy, and left-sided heart failure.

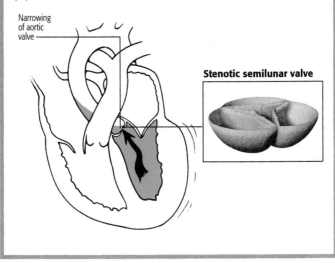

Narrowing of aortic valve

**Stenotic semilunar valve**

## *Causes*

- ◆ Idiopathic fibrosis and calcification
- ◆ Congenital aortic bicuspid valve
- ◆ Rheumatic fever
- ◆ Atherosclerosis

## ▲ *Pathophysiologic changes*

Abnormal diastolic function ➡️    **Exertional dyspnea**

Increased oxygen requirement    **Angina**
by hypertrophic myocardium
and diminished oxygen delivery
secondary to compression of
coronary vessels ➡️

Systemic vasodilation or arrhyth-    **Syncope**
mias ➡️

Left-sided heart failure ➡️    **Pulmonary congestion**

Forced blood flow across stenotic    **Harsh, rasping, crescendo-**
valve ➡️    **decrescendo systolic murmur**

## ▲ *Management*

- ◆ Periodic noninvasive evaluation — *to monitor severity of valve narrowing*
- ◆ Cardiac glycosides — *to control atrial fibrillation*
- ◆ Low-sodium diet, diuretics — *to treat left-sided heart failure*
- ◆ Prophylactic antibiotics before and after surgery or dental care — *to prevent endocarditis*
- ◆ Percutaneous balloon aortic valvuloplasty — *to reduce degree of stenosis*
- ◆ Aortic valve replacement — *to replace diseased valve*

# Cardiomyopathy, dilated

◆ Disease of heart muscle fibers
◆ Usually not diagnosed until advanced stage; prognosis generally poor

**THE PATHO PICTURE**

## UNDERSTANDING
## DILATED CARDIOMYOPATHY

Extensively damaged myocardial muscle fibers reduce contractility of the left ventricle. As systolic function declines, stroke volume, ejection fraction, and cardiac output fall. The sympathetic nervous system is stimulated to increase heart rate and contractility. The kidneys are stimulated to retain sodium and water to maintain cardiac output, and vasoconstriction also occurs as the renin-angiotensin system is stimulated.

When compensatory mechanisms can no longer maintain cardiac output, the heart begins to fail. Left ventricular dilation occurs as venous return and systemic vascular resistance rise. Eventually, the atria also dilate as more work is required to pump blood into the full ventricles. Cardiomegaly occurs as a consequence of dilation of the atria and ventricles.

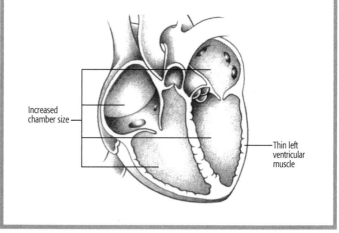

Increased chamber size

Thin left ventricular muscle

## Causes

◆ Viral or bacterial infections
◆ Hypertension
◆ Peripartum syndrome related to toxemia
◆ Ischemic heart disease
◆ Valvular disease
◆ Drug hypersensitivity
◆ Chemotherapy
◆ Cardiotoxic effects of drug or alcohol

## ◣ *Pathophysiologic changes*

| | |
|---|---|
| Left-sided heart failure ➡ | Shortness of breath, orthopnea, dyspnea on exertion, paroxysmal nocturnal dyspnea, fatigue, dry cough at night |
| Right-sided heart failure ➡ | Peripheral edema, hepatomegaly, jugular venous distention, weight gain |
| Low cardiac output ➡ | Peripheral cyanosis, tachycardia |
| Mitral and tricuspid insufficiency secondary to cardiomegaly and weak papillary muscles ➡ | Pansystolic murmur |
| Heart failure ➡ | S3 and S4 gallop rhythms |
| Atrial fibrillation ➡ | Irregular pulse |
| Decreased cardiac output ➡ | Decreased renal perfusion |

## ▲▲▲ *Management*

- ◆ Angiotensin-converting enzyme (ACE) inhibitors — *to reduce afterload through vasodilation*
- ◆ Diuretics — *to reduce fluid retention* (for patient who doesn't respond, digoxin — *to improve myocardial contractility*)
- ◆ Hydralazine and isosorbide dinitrate — *to produce vasodilation*
- ◆ Beta-adrenergic blockers — *to treat New York Heart Association (NYHA) class II or III heart failure*
- ◆ Antiarrhythmics or implantable cardioverter-defibrillator (ICD) — *to control arrhythmias*
- ◆ Pacemaker insertion — *to correct arrhythmias*
- ◆ Biventricular pacemaker — *for cardiac resynchronization therapy* (if symptoms continue despite optimal drug therapy, QRS duration is 0.13 second or more, or ejection fraction is 35% or less, patient is classified as NYHA class III or IV heart failure)
- ◆ Revascularization (such as coronary artery bypass graft surgery) — *to manage dilated cardiomyopathy from ischemia*
- ◆ Valvular repair or replacement — *to manage dilated cardiomyopathy from valve dysfunction*
- ◆ Heart transplantation — *for patient refractory to medical therapy*
- ◆ Lifestyle modifications (smoking cessation; low-fat, low-sodium diet; physical activity; abstinence from alcohol) — *to reduce symptoms and improve quality of life*

# Cardiomyopathy, hypertrophic obstructive

◆ Primary disease of cardiac muscle
◆ 50% of all sudden deaths in competitive athletes are due to HOCM

**THE PATHO PICTURE**

### UNDERSTANDING HYPERTROPHIC OBSTRUCTIVE CARDIOMYOPATHY

Hypertrophic obstructive cardiomyopathy (HOCM) affects diastolic function. The left ventricle and intraventricular septum hypertrophy and become stiff, non-compliant, and unable to relax during ventricular filling. Ventricular filling decreases and left ventricular filling pressure rises, causing a rise in left atrial and pulmonary venous pressures. This leads to rapid, forceful contractions of the left ventricle and impaired relaxation. The forceful ejection of blood draws the anterior leaflet of the mitral valve to the intraventricular septum. This causes early closure of the outflow tract, decreasing ejection fraction.

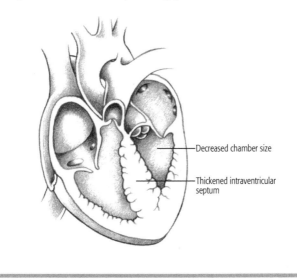

Decreased chamber size

Thickened intraventricular septum

## *Cause*

◆ Autosomal dominant trait

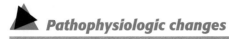

## *Pathophysiologic changes*

| | |
|---|---|
| Mitral insufficiency ➡ | **Systolic ejection murmur along left sternal border and at apex** |
| Inability of intramural coronary arteries to supply enough blood to meet increased oxygen demands of hypertrophied heart ➡ | **Angina** |
| Arrhythmias or reduced ventricular filling leading to reduced cardiac output ➡ | **Syncope** |
| Worsening of outflow tract obstruction from exercise-induced catecholamine release ➡ | **Activity intolerance** |
| Vigorous left ventricular contractions and early termination of left ventricular ejection ➡ | **Abrupt arterial pulse** |
| Enlarged atrium ➡ | **Irregular pulse (atrial fibrillation)** |

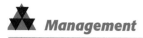 *Management*

- ◆ Beta-adrenergic blockers — *to slow heart rate, reduce myocardial oxygen demands, and increase ventricular filling by relaxing obstructing muscle, thereby increasing cardiac output*
- ◆ Antiarrhythmic drugs, such as amiodarone — *to reduce arrhythmias*
- ◆ Cardioversion — *to treat atrial fibrillation*
- ◆ Anticoagulation — *to reduce risk of systemic embolism with atrial fibrillation*
- ◆ Verapamil or diltiazem — *to reduce septal stiffness and elevated diastolic pressures*
- ◆ Implantable cardioverter-defibrillator (ICD) — *to treat ventricular arrhythmias*
- ◆ Ventricular myotomy or myectomy (resection of hypertrophied septum) — *to ease outflow tract obstruction and relieve symptoms*

# Cardiomyopathy, restrictive

◆ Disease of heart muscle fibers
◆ Irreversible if severe

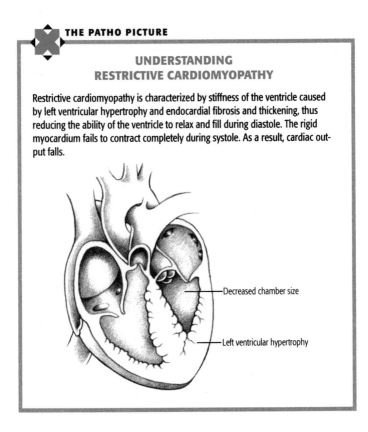

**THE PATHO PICTURE**

### UNDERSTANDING
### RESTRICTIVE CARDIOMYOPATHY

Restrictive cardiomyopathy is characterized by stiffness of the ventricle caused by left ventricular hypertrophy and endocardial fibrosis and thickening, thus reducing the ability of the ventricle to relax and fill during diastole. The rigid myocardium fails to contract completely during systole. As a result, cardiac output falls.

Decreased chamber size

Left ventricular hypertrophy

## *Causes*

◆ Amyloidosis
◆ Sarcoidosis
◆ Hemochromomatosis
◆ Infiltrative neoplastic disease

## *Pathophysiologic changes*

| | |
|---|---|
| Heart failure ➤ | Fatigue, dyspnea, orthopnea, chest pain, edema, liver engorgement, peripheral cyanosis, pallor, and S3 or S4 gallop rhythms |
| Mitral and tricuspid insufficiency ➤ | Systolic murmurs |

## *Management*

◆ Deferoxamine — *to bind iron in restrictive cardiomyopathy due to hemochromatosis*
◆ Digoxin, diuretics, and restricted sodium diet — *to ease symptoms of heart failure*
◆ Oral vasodilators — *to decrease afterload and facilitate ventricular ejection*

# Heart failure

◆ Syndrome that occurs when heart can't pump enough blood to meet body's metabolic needs
◆ Results in intravascular and interstitial volume overload and poor tissue perfusion
◆ May be classified according to side of heart affected (left- or right-sided heart failure) or cardiac cycle involved (systolic or diastolic dysfunction)

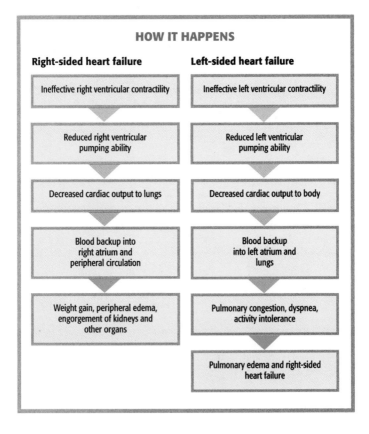

**HOW IT HAPPENS**

| Right-sided heart failure | Left-sided heart failure |
|---|---|
| Ineffective right ventricular contractility | Ineffective left ventricular contractility |
| Reduced right ventricular pumping ability | Reduced left ventricular pumping ability |
| Decreased cardiac output to lungs | Decreased cardiac output to body |
| Blood backup into right atrium and peripheral circulation | Blood backup into left atrium and lungs |
| Weight gain, peripheral edema, engorgement of kidneys and other organs | Pulmonary congestion, dyspnea, activity intolerance |
| | Pulmonary edema and right-sided heart failure |

## *Causes*

◆ Abnormal cardiac muscle function
◆ Abnormal left ventricular volume, pressure, or filling

# ▲ *Pathophysiologic changes*

### LEFT-SIDED HEART FAILURE

Pulmonary congestion ➡️

Dyspnea, orthopnea, paroxysmal nocturnal dyspnea, nonproductive cough, crackles

Reduced oxygenation; inability to increase cardiac output in response to physical activity ➡️

Fatigue

Left ventricular hypertrophy ➡️

Point of maximal impulse displaced toward left anterior axillary line

Sympathetic stimulation ➡️

Tachycardia

Rapid ventricular filling ➡️

$S_3$

Atrial contraction against noncompliant ventricle ➡️

$S_4$

Peripheral vasoconstriction ➡️

Cool, pale skin

### RIGHT-SIDED HEART FAILURE

Venous congestion ➡️

Elevated jugular vein distention, positive hepatojugular reflux, and hepatomegaly

Liver engorgement ➡️

Right upper quadrant pain

Congestion of liver and intestines ➡️

Anorexia, fullness, and nausea

Nocturnal fluid redistribution and reabsorption ➡️

Nocturia

Fluid volume excess ➡️

Weight gain, edema

Fluid retention ➡️

Ascites or anasarca

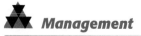 *Management*

- Angiotensin-converting enzyme (ACE) inhibitors for patients with left ventricle dysfunction — *to reduce preload and afterload*
- Digoxin — *to increase myocardial contractility, improve cardiac output, reduce ventricular volume, and decrease ventricular stretch*
- Diuretics — *to reduce fluid volume overload and venous return*
- Beta-adrenergic blockers in patient with New York Heart Association class II or III heart failure caused by left ventricular systolic dysfunction — *to prevent remodeling*
- Inotropic therapy with dobutamine or milrinone — *for acute treatment of heart failure exacerbation*
- Diuretics, nitrates, morphine, and oxygen — *to treat pulmonary edema*
- Lifestyle modifications (exercise; weight loss; reduced sodium, alcohol, and fat intake; smoking cessation; stress reduction) — *to reduce symptoms of heart failure*
- Coronary artery bypass surgery or angioplasty — *for heart failure due to CAD*
- Heart transplantation — *for patient receiving aggressive medical treatment but still experiencing limitations or repeated hospitalizations*

# Hypertension

◆ Intermittent or sustained elevation of systolic blood pressure > 139 mm Hg or diastolic blood pressure > 89 mm Hg

◆ Occurs as two major types: essential (primary) hypertension and secondary hypertension

**✖ THE PATHO PICTURE**

## UNDERSTANDING HYPERTENSION

Arterial blood pressure is a product of total peripheral resistance (TPR) and cardiac output (CO). CO is increased by conditions that increase heart rate, stroke volume, or both. TPR is increased by factors that increase blood viscosity or reduce the lumen size of vessels, especially the arterioles.

Several theories help explain how hypertension develops, including:

◆ changes in the arteriolar bed, causing increased TPR

◆ abnormally increased tone in the sympathetic nervous system, causing increased TPR

◆ increased blood volume resulting from renal or hormonal dysfunction

◆ increased arteriolar thickening caused by genetic factors, leading to increased TPR

◆ abnormal renin release, resulting in formation of angiotensin II, which constricts the arteriole and increases blood volume.

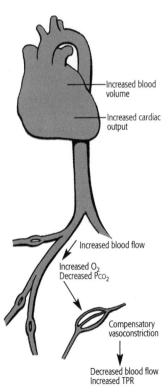

Increased blood volume

Increased cardiac output

Increased blood flow

Increased $O_2$
Decreased $P_{CO_2}$

Compensatory vasoconstriction

Decreased blood flow
Increased TPR

## *Causes*

### PRIMARY HYPERTENSION
◆ Unknown

### SECONDARY HYPERTENSION
◆ Renal artery stenosis and parenchymal disease
◆ Brain tumor, quadriplegia, and head injury
◆ Pheochromocytoma, Cushing's syndrome, hyperaldosteronism, and thyroid, pituitary, or parathyroid dysfunction
◆ Oral contraceptives, cocaine, epoetin alfa, sympathetic stimulants, monoamine oxidase inhibitors taken with tyramine, estrogen replacement therapy, and nonsteroidal anti-inflammatory drugs

## *Risk factors*

### PRIMARY HYPERTENSION
◆ Family history; advancing age
◆ Obesity; sedentary lifestyle
◆ Tobacco use; high intake of sodium, saturated fat, alcohol
◆ Stress
◆ Diabetes mellitus

# ▲ *Pathophysiologic changes*

Vasoconstriction ■▶ **Elevated blood pressure**

Stenosis or aneurysm ■▶ **Bruits (may be heard over abdominal aorta or carotid, renal, and femoral arteries)**

Decreased tissue perfusion due to vasoconstriction of blood vessels ■▶ **Dizziness, confusion, and fatigue**

Retinal damage ■▶ **Blurry vision**

Increased blood flow to kidneys; increased glomerular filtration ■▶ **Nocturia**

Increased capillary pressure ■▶ **Edema**

# ▲ *Management*

- ◆ Lifestyle modifications (exercise; weight loss; reduced sodium, alcohol, and fat intake; smoking cessation; stress reduction) — *to reduce symptoms of hypertension*
- ◆ Drug therapy (thiazide-type diuretic, ACE inhibitor, angiotensin receptor blocker, beta-adrenergic blocker, calcium channel blocker, or combination) — *to treat primary hypertension*
- ◆ Correction of underlying cause and control of hypertensive effects — *to treat secondary hypertension*

# Mitral insufficiency

◆ Inadequate closing of mitral valve
◆ Backflow of blood from left ventricle to right atrium during systole

**THE PATHO PICTURE**

## UNDERSTANDING MITRAL INSUFFICIENCY

An abnormality of the mitral leaflets, mitral annulus, chordae tendineae, papillary muscles, left atrium, or left ventricle can lead to mitral insufficiency. Blood from the left ventricle flows back into the left atrium during systole; the atrium enlarges to accommodate the backflow. As a result, the left ventricle also dilates to accommodate the increased blood volume from the atrium and to compensate for diminishing cardiac output. Ventricular hypertrophy and increased end-diastolic pressure result in increased pulmonary artery pressure, eventually leading to left-sided and right-sided heart failure.

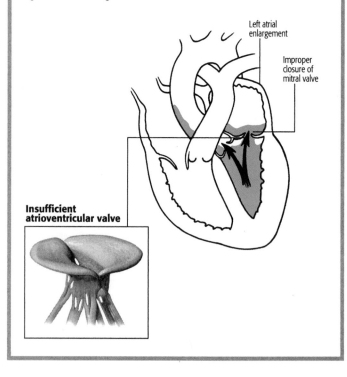

Left atrial enlargement

Improper closure of mitral valve

**Insufficient atrioventricular valve**

## *Causes*

◆ Rheumatic fever
◆ Mitral valve prolapse
◆ Hypertrophic obstructive cardiomyopathy
◆ Myocardial infarction
◆ Ruptured chordae tendineae
◆ Transposition of great arteries

## ◢ *Pathophysiologic changes*

| | |
|---|---|
| Left ventricular dysfunction ➡ | **Orthopnea, dyspnea, fatigue, peripheral edema, jugular venous distention, tachycardia, crackles, pulmonary edema** |
| Inadequate coronary artery circulation ➡ | **Angina** |
| Regurgitant blood flow ➡ | **Holosystolic murmur at apex** |

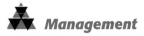

## Management

- Digoxin, low-sodium diet, diuretics, vasodilators, and especially angiotensin-converting enzyme inhibitors — *to treat left-sided heart failure*
- Oxygen (in acute situations) — *to increase oxygenation*
- Anticoagulants — *to prevent thrombus formation around diseased or replaced valves*
- Prophylactic antibiotics before and after surgery or dental care — *to prevent endocarditis*
- Nitroglycerin — *to relieve angina*
- Annuloplasty or valvuloplasty — *to reconstruct or repair damaged valve*
- Prosthetic valve — *to replace damaged valve that can't be repaired*

# Mitral stenosis

◆ Narrowing of mitral valve orifice
◆ Valve leaflets thickened by fibrosis and calcification

**THE PATHO PICTURE**

### UNDERSTANDING MITRAL STENOSIS

Narrowing of the valve by valvular abnormalities, fibrosis, or calcification obstructs blood flow from the left atrium to the left ventricle. Left atrial volume and pressure rise and the chamber dilates. Greater resistance to blood flow causes pulmonary hypertension, right ventricular hypertrophy, and right-sided heart failure. Inadequate filling of the left ventricle results in low cardiac output.

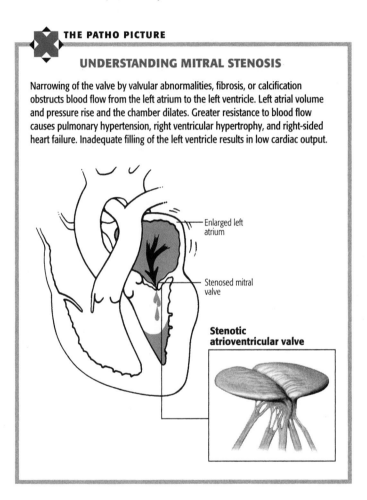

Enlarged left atrium

Stenosed mitral valve

**Stenotic atrioventricular valve**

## *Causes*

- ◆ Rheumatic fever
- ◆ Congenital abnormalities
- ◆ Atrial myxoma
- ◆ Endocarditis
- ◆ Adverse effect of fenfluramine and phentermine diet drug combination

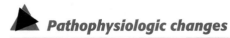 *Pathophysiologic changes*

| | |
|---|---|
| Cardiac dysfunction ▶ | Dyspnea on exertion, paroxysmal noctural dyspnea, orthopnea, weakness, fatigue, and palpitations |
| Heart failure ▶ | Peripheral edema, jugular venous distention, hepatomegaly, tachycardia, crackles, pulmonary edema |
| Turbulent blood flow over stenotic valve ▶ | Opening snap and diastolic murmur |

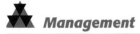

## Management

- Digoxin, low-sodium diet, diuretics, vasodilators, and especially ACE inhibitors — *to treat left-sided heart failure*
- Oxygen (in acute situations) — *to increase oxygenation*
- Anticoagulants — *to prevent thrombus formation around diseased or replaced valves*
- Prophylactic antibiotics before and after surgery or dental care — *to prevent endocarditis*
- Nitrates — *to relieve angina*
- Beta-adrenergic blockers or digoxin — *to slow ventricular rate in atrial fibrillation or atrial flutter*
- Cardioversion — *to convert atrial fibrillation to sinus rhythm*
- Balloon valvuloplasty — *to enlarge orifice of stenotic mitral valve*
- Prosthetic valve — *to replace damaged valve that can't be repaired*

# Pericarditis

◆ Inflammation of pericardium
◆ Can be fibrous or effusive, with purulent, serous, or hemorrhagic exudate (acute pericarditis)
◆ Is characterized by dense, fibrous pericardial thickening (chronic constrictive pericarditis)

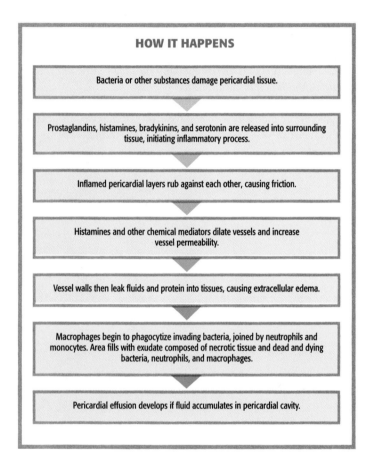

**HOW IT HAPPENS**

Bacteria or other substances damage pericardial tissue.

Prostaglandins, histamines, bradykinins, and serotonin are released into surrounding tissue, initiating inflammatory process.

Inflamed pericardial layers rub against each other, causing friction.

Histamines and other chemical mediators dilate vessels and increase vessel permeability.

Vessel walls then leak fluids and protein into tissues, causing extracellular edema.

Macrophages begin to phagocytize invading bacteria, joined by neutrophils and monocytes. Area fills with exudate composed of necrotic tissue and dead and dying bacteria, neutrophils, and macrophages.

Pericardial effusion develops if fluid accumulates in pericardial cavity.

## *Causes*

◆ Bacterial, fungal, or viral infection (infectious pericarditis)
◆ Neoplasms
◆ High-dose radiation to chest
◆ Uremia
◆ Hypersensitivity or autoimmune disease
◆ Cardiac injury, cardiac surgery
◆ Drugs, such as hydralazine or procainamide
◆ Idiopathic factors (most common in acute pericarditis)

## ▲ *Pathophysiologic changes*

| | |
|---|---|
| Roughened, inflamed, irritated pericardial membranes ➡ | **Pericardial friction rub; sharp, typically sudden pain, usually starting over sternum and radiating to neck, shoulders, back, and arms** |
| Pleuritic pain ➡ | **Shallow, rapid respirations** |
| Inflammation ➡ | **Mild fever** |
| Pericardial effusion ➡ | **Dyspnea, orthopnea, tachycardia, and other signs of heart failure** |
| Fluid buildup ➡ | **Muffled and distant heart sounds** |
| Increased systemic venous pressure ➡ | **Fluid retention, ascites, hepatomegaly, jugular venous distention, and other signs of chronic right-sided heart failure** |

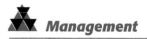

## *Management*

- ◆ Bed rest as long as fever and pain persist — *to reduce metabolic needs*
- ◆ Nonsteroidal anti-inflammatory drugs (NSAIDs), such as aspirin and indomethacin — *to relieve pain and reduce inflammation*
- ◆ Corticosteroids — *if NSAIDs are ineffective and no infection exists*
- ◆ Antibacterial, antifungal, or antiviral therapy — *if infectious cause is suspected*
- ◆ Pericardiocentesis — *to remove excess fluid from pericardial space*
- ◆ Partial pericardectomy — *to create window that allows fluid to drain into pleural space (recurrent pericarditis)*
- ◆ Total pericardectomy — *to permit adequate filling and contraction of heart (constrictive pericarditis)*

# Shock, cardiogenic

◆ Condition of diminished cardiac output that severely impairs tissue perfusion
◆ Sometimes called pump failure

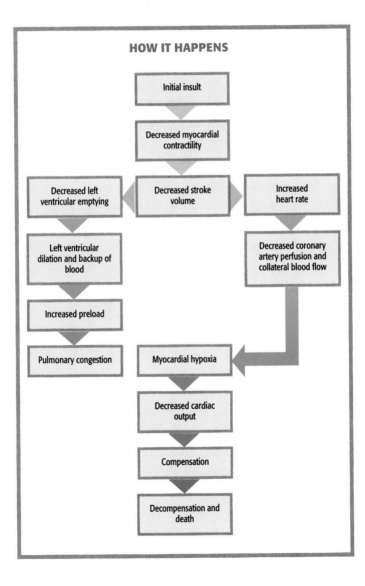

## *Causes*

- Myocardial infarction
- Myocardial ischemia
- Papillary muscle dysfunction
- End-stage cardiomyopathy
- Myocarditis
- Acute mitral or aortic insufficiency
- Ventricular septal defect
- Ventricular aneurysm

## ▲ *Pathophysiologic changes*

| | |
|---|---|
| Sympathetic stimulation ➡ | **Tachycardia, bounding pulse** |
| Cerebral hypoxia ➡ | **Restlessness, irritability, tachypnea** |
| Vasoconstriction ➡ | **Reduced urine output; cool, pale skin** |
| Failure of compensatory mechanisms ➡ | **Hypotension** |
| Reduced stroke volume, decreased cardiac output ➡ | **Narrowed pulse pressure; weak, rapid, thready pulse** |
| Poor renal perfusion ➡ | **Reduced urine output** |
| Hypoxia ➡ | **Cyanosis** |
| Reduced cerebral perfusion, acid-base imbalance, or electrolyte abnormalities ➡ | **Unconsciousness and absent reflexes** |
| Weakening of patient; respiratory center depression ➡ | **Slow, shallow, or Cheyne-Stokes respirations** |

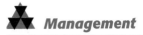 *Management*

- Maintenance of patent airway; preparation for intubation and mechanical ventilation — *to prevent or manage respiratory distress*
- Supplemental oxygen — *to increase oxygenation*
- I.V. fluids, crystalloids, colloids, or blood products, as necessary — *to maintain intravascular volume*
- Inotropic drugs — *to increase heart contractility and cardiac output*
- Vasodilators given with vasopressor — *to reduce left ventricle's workload*
- Intra-aortic balloon pump (IABP) therapy — *to reduce left ventricle's workload by decreasing systemic vascular resistance*
- Coronary artery revascularization — *to restore coronary artery blood flow if cardiogenic shock is due to acute MI*
- Emergency surgery — *to repair papillary muscle rupture or ventricular septal defect if either is cause of cardiogenic shock*
- Ventricular assist device — *to assist pumping action of heart when IABP and drug therapy fail*

# Shock, hypovolemic

◆ Reduced intravascular blood volume causes circulatory dysfunction and inadequate tissue perfusion
◆ Requires early recognition and prompt treatment to improve prognosis

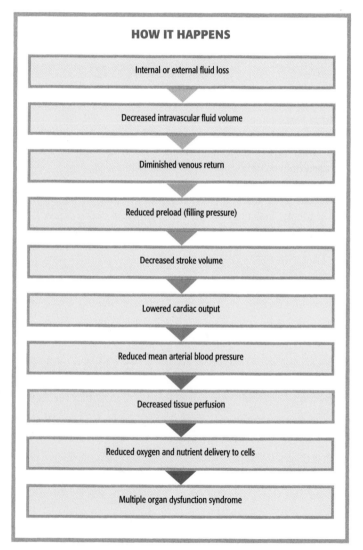

**HOW IT HAPPENS**

Internal or external fluid loss

Decreased intravascular fluid volume

Diminished venous return

Reduced preload (filling pressure)

Decreased stroke volume

Lowered cardiac output

Reduced mean arterial blood pressure

Decreased tissue perfusion

Reduced oxygen and nutrient delivery to cells

Multiple organ dysfunction syndrome

## *Causes*

◆ Blood loss
◆ GI fluid loss
◆ Burns
◆ Renal loss (diabetic ketoacidosis, diabetes insipidus, adrenal insufficiency)
◆ Fluid shifts
◆ Ascites
◆ Peritonitis
◆ Hemothorax

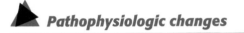 *Pathophysiologic changes*

| | |
|---|---|
| Sympathetic stimulation ➡ | Tachycardia |
| Cerebral hypoxia ➡ | Restlessness, irritability, and tachypnea |
| Reduced fluid volume; vasoconstriction ➡ | Reduced urine output; cool, pale, clammy skin |
| Failure of compensatory mechanisms ➡ | Hypotension |
| Reduced stroke volume; decreased cardiac output ➡ | Narrowed pulse pressure; weak, rapid, thready pulse |
| Weakening of patient ➡ | Shallow respirations |
| Poor renal perfusion ➡ | Reduced urine output |
| Hypoxia ➡ | Cyanosis |
| Tissue anoxia ➡ | Metabolic acidosis |

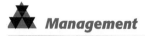 *Management*

- ◆ Maintenance of patent airway; preparation for intubation and mechanical ventilation — *to prevent or manage respiratory distress*
- ◆ Supplemental oxygen — *to increase oxygenation*
- ◆ Pneumatic antishock garment — *to control internal and external hemorrhage by direct pressure*
- ◆ Fluids, such as normal saline or lactated Ringer's solution — *to restore filling pressures*
- ◆ Packed red blood cells — *to restore blood loss and improve blood's oxygen-carrying capacity (hemorrhagic shock)*

# Shock, septic

- Inadequate tissue perfusion, metabolic changes, and circulatory collapse as response to infection
- Developed by 25% of patients with gram-negative bacteremia

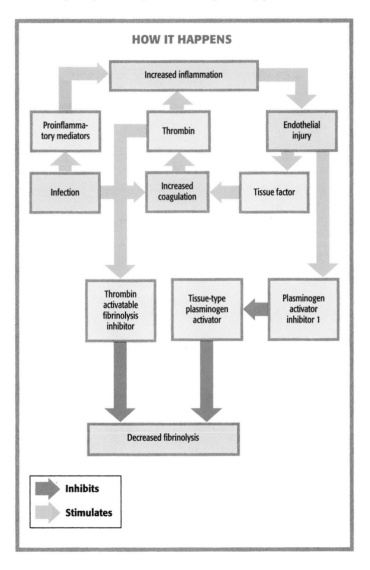

**HOW IT HAPPENS**

Increased inflammation

Proinflamma-tory mediators

Thrombin

Endothelial injury

Infection

Increased coagulation

Tissue factor

Thrombin activatable fibrinolysis inhibitor

Tissue-type plasminogen activator

Plasminogen activator inhibitor 1

Decreased fibrinolysis

Inhibits

Stimulates

## *Causes*

◆ Gram-negative bacteria
◆ Gram-positive bacteria

### ▲ *Pathophysiologic changes*

| | |
|---|---|
| Infection ➡ | **Chills and fever** |
| Sympathetic stimulation ➡ | **Tachycardia and bounding pulse** |
| Cerebral hypoxia ➡ | **Restlessness, irritability, tachypnea** |
| Vasoconstriction ➡ | **Reduced urine output** |
| Vasodilation ➡ | **Warm, dry skin** |
| Failure of compensatory mechanisms ➡ | **Hypotension** |
| Hypoxia ➡ | **Cyanosis** |
| Reduced cerebral perfusion, acid-base imbalance, or electrolyte abnormalities ➡ | **Unconsciousness and absent reflexes** |
| Decompensation ➡ | **Rapidly falling blood pressure** |
| Respiratory center depression ➡ | **Slow, shallow, or Cheyne-Stokes respirations** |

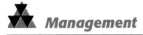 *Management*

- ◆ Antibiotic therapy — *to eradicate causative organism*
- ◆ Inotropic and vasopressor drugs, such as dopamine, dobutamine, and norepinephrine — *to improve perfusion and maintain blood pressure*
- ◆ Maintenance of patent airway; preparation for intubation and mechanical ventilation — *to prevent or manage respiratory distress*
- ◆ Supplemental oxygen — *to increase oxygenation*
- ◆ I.V. fluids, crystalloids, colloids, or blood products, as necessary — *to maintain intravascular volume*
- ◆ Monoclonal antibodies to tumor necrosis factor, endotoxin, and interleukin-1 — *to counteract septic shock mediators* (investigational)

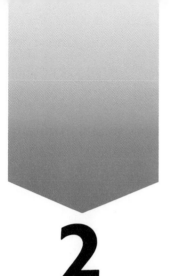

# 2

# Respiratory disorders

# PATHOPHYSIOLOGIC CONCEPTS

## *Atelectasis*

♦ Occurs when alveolar sacs or entire lung segments expand incompletely, producing partial or complete lung collapse
♦ Removes certain lung regions from gas exchange, allowing unoxygenated blood to pass unchanged through these regions, resulting in hypoxia
♦ May be chronic or acute; commonly occurs in patients undergoing upper abdominal or thoracic surgery

## *Bronchiectasis*

♦ Chronic abnormal dilation of bronchi and destruction of bronchial walls, which can occur throughout tracheobronchial tree
♦ May also be confined to single segment or lobe
♦ Usually bilateral in nature, involving basilar segments of lower lobes
♦ Three forms of bronchiectasis: cylindrical, fusiform (varicose), and saccular (cystic)

### FORMS OF BRONCHIECTASIS

Bronchiectasis occurs in three forms: cylindrical, fusiform (varicose), and saccular (cystic). In cylindrical bronchiectasis, bronchioles are usually symmetrically dilated, whereas in fusiform bronchiectasis, bronchioles are deformed. In saccular bronchiectasis, large bronchi become enlarged and balloonlike.

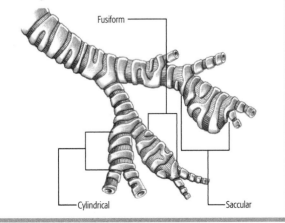

- Results from conditions associated with repeated damage to bronchial walls with abnormal mucociliary clearance, which causes breakdown of supporting tissue adjacent to airways
- Sputum stagnates in dilated bronchi and leads to secondary infection, characterized by inflammation and leukocytic accumulations
- Additional debris collects within and occludes bronchi
- Increasing pressure from retained secretions induces mucosal injury

## Cyanosis

- Bluish discoloration of skin and mucous membranes; may be central or peripheral
  – central cyanosis: decreased oxygen saturation of hemoglobin in arterial blood; best observed in buccal mucous membranes and lips
  – peripheral cyanosis: slowed blood circulation of fingers and toes; best visualized by examining nail bed area
- Caused by desaturation with oxygen or reduced hemoglobin amounts (develops when 5 g of hemoglobin is desaturated, even if hemoglobin counts are adequate or reduced)

## Hypoxemia

- Reduced oxygenation of arterial blood, evidenced by reduced $Pao_2$ of arterial blood gases
- Can be caused by decreased oxygen content of inspired gas, hypoventilation, diffusion abnormalities, abnormal $\dot{V}/\dot{Q}$ ratios, and pulmonary right-to-left shunts
- Variable physiologic mechanism for each cause
- Can lead to tissue hypoxia
- Can occur anywhere in body

# DISORDERS

## Acute respiratory distress syndrome (ARDS)

◆ Form of pulmonary edema that can quickly lead to acute respiratory failure

◆ Also known as shock lung, stiff lung, white lung, wet lung

◆ Diagnosis is difficult; death can occur within 48 hours if not promptly diagnosed and treated

**THE PATHO PICTURE**

### UNDERSTANDING ARDS

In phase 1, injury reduces normal blood flow to the lungs. Platelets aggregate and release histamine (H), serotonin (S), and bradykinin (B).

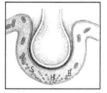

In phase 2, the released substances inflame and damage the alveolar capillary membrane, increasing capillary permeability. Fluids then shift into the interstitial space.

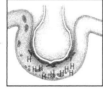

In phase 3, capillary permeability increases and proteins and fluids leak out, increasing interstitial osmotic pressure and causing pulmonary edema.

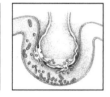

In phase 4, decreased blood flow and fluids in the alveoli damage surfactant and impair the cell's ability to produce more. The alveoli then collapse, impairing gas exchange.

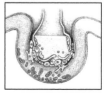

In phase 5, oxygenation is impaired, but carbon dioxide ($CO_2$) easily crosses the alveolar capillary membrane and is expired. Blood oxygen ($O_2$) and $CO_2$ levels are low.

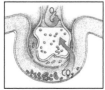

In phase 6, pulmonary edema worsens and inflammation leads to fibrosis. Gas exchange is further impeded.

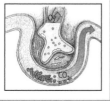

## *Causes*

◆ Indirect or direct lung trauma
◆ Anaphylaxis
◆ Aspiration of gastric contents
◆ Diffuse pneumonia (especially viral)
◆ Drug overdose
◆ Idiosyncratic drug reaction
◆ Inhalation of noxious gases (nitrous oxide, ammonia, chlorine)
◆ Near drowning
◆ Oxygen toxicity
◆ Sepsis

## ▲ *Pathophysiologic changes*

| | |
|---|---|
| Decreasing oxygen levels in blood ➡ | **Tachycardia; rapid, shallow breathing; dyspnea** |
| Hypoxemia and its effects on pneumotaxic center ➡ | **Increased rate of ventilation** |
| Increased effort required to expand stiff lung ➡ | **Intercostal and suprasternal retractions** |
| Fluid accumulation in lungs ➡ | **Crackles and rhonchi** |
| Hypoxic brain cells ➡ | **Restlessness, apprehension, mental sluggishness, and motor dysfunction** |
| Accumulation of carbon dioxide in blood ➡ | **Respiratory acidosis** |
| Failure of compensatory mechanisms ➡ | **Metabolic acidosis** |

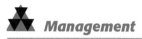 *Management*

♦ Administration of humidified oxygen, ventilatory support with intubation, volume ventilation, and positive end-expiratory pressure — *to improve oxygenation*
♦ Sedatives, narcotics, or neuromuscular blockers during mechanical ventilation — *to minimize restlessness, oxygen consumption, and carbon dioxide production and to facilitate ventilation*
♦ Sodium bicarbonate — *to reverse severe metabolic acidosis*
♦ I.V. fluid administration — *to maintain blood pressure by treating hypovolemia*
♦ Vasopressors — *to maintain blood pressure*
♦ Antimicrobial drugs — *to treat nonviral infections*
♦ Diuretics — *to reduce interstitial and pulmonary edema*
♦ Correction of electrolyte and acid-base imbalances — *to maintain cellular integrity (particularly sodium-potassium pump)*
♦ Fluid restriction — *to prevent increased interstitial and alveolar edema*

# Asthma

- Chronic inflammatory airway disorder characterized by airflow obstruction and airway hyperresponsiveness to multiplicity of stimuli
- Type of chronic obstructive pulmonary disease (COPD)
- May result from sensitivity to extrinsic or intrinsic allergens

**THE PATHO PICTURE**

## UNDERSTANDING ASTHMA

In asthma, hyperresponsiveness of the airways and bronchospasms occur. These illustrations show how an asthma attack progresses.

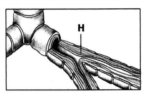

- Histamine (H) attaches to receptor sites in larger bronchi, causing swelling of the smooth muscles.

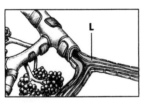

- Leukotrienes (L) attach to receptor sites in the smaller bronchi and cause swelling of smooth muscle there. Leukotrienes also cause prostaglandins to travel through the bloodstream to the lungs, where they enhance histamine's effects.

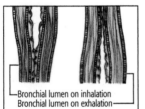

Bronchial lumen on inhalation
Bronchial lumen on exhalation

- Histamine stimulates the mucous membranes to secrete excessive mucus, further narrowing the bronchial lumen. On inhalation, the narrowed bronchial lumen can still expand slightly; on exhalation, however, the increased intrathoracic pressure closes the bronchial lumen completely.

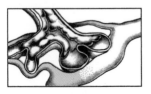

- Mucus fills lung bases, inhibiting alveolar ventilation. Blood is shunted to alveoli in other parts of the lungs, but it still can't compensate for diminished ventilation.

## *Causes*

◆ Extrinsic asthma: pollen, animal dander, house dust or mold, kapok or feather pillows, food additives containing sulfites, other sensitizing substances
◆ Intrinsic asthma: irritants, emotional stress, fatigue, endocrine changes, temperature variations, humidity variations, exposure to noxious fumes, anxiety, coughing or laughing, genetic factors

### ◢ *Pathophysiologic changes*

| | |
|---|---|
| Bronchial constriction ➧ | Sudden dyspnea, wheezing, tightness in chest, diminished breath sounds |
| Excessive mucus production ➧ | Coughing; thick, clear, or yellow sputum |
| Hypoxemia ➧ | Rapid pulse, tachypnea, use of accessory respiratory muscles |

# ▲▲▲ *Management*

- ◆ Identification and avoidance of precipitating factors (environmental allergens or irritants) — *to prevent asthma attacks*
- ◆ Desensitization to specific antigens — *to decrease severity of asthma attacks during future exposure to allergen*
- ◆ Bronchodilators — *to decrease bronchoconstriction, reduce bronchial airway edema, and increase pulmonary ventilation*
- ◆ Corticosteroids — *to decrease inflammation and edema of airways*
- ◆ Mast cell stabilizers — *to block acute obstructive effects of antigen exposure (inhibit degranulation of mast cells, thereby preventing release of chemical mediators responsible for anaphylaxis)*
- ◆ Leukotriene modifiers and leukotriene receptor antagonists (may be used as adjunctive therapy to avoid high-dose inhaled corticosteroids or when patient is noncompliant with corticosteroid therapy) — *to inhibit potent bronchoconstriction and inflammatory effects of cysteinyl leukotrienes*
- ◆ Anticholinergic bronchodilators — *to block acetylcholine (another chemical mediator)*
- ◆ Low-flow humidified oxygen (amount delivered should maintain $Pao_2$ between 65 and 85 mm Hg, as determined by ABG analysis) — *to treat dyspnea, cyanosis, and hypoxemia*
- ◆ Mechanical ventilation — *if patient fails to respond to initial ventilatory support and drugs, or develops respiratory failure*
- ◆ Relaxation exercises (yoga) — *to increase circulation and help patient recover from asthma attack*

# Chronic bronchitis

- Form of chronic obstructive pulmonary disease (COPD)
- Characterized by excessive production of tracheobronchial mucus and chronic cough (at least 3 months each year for 2 consecutive years)
- Distinguishing characteristic is airflow obstruction

**THE PATHO PICTURE**

## UNDERSTANDING CHRONIC BRONCHITIS

In chronic bronchitis, irritants inflame the tracheobronchial tree over time, leading to increased mucus production and a narrowed or blocked airway. As the inflammation continues, goblet and epithelial cells hypertrophy. Because the natural defense mechanisms are blocked, the airways accumulate debris in the respiratory tract.

**Cross section of normal bronchial tube**

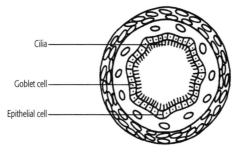

**Narrowed bronchial tube in chronic bronchitis**

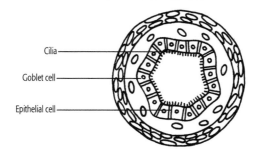

## *Causes*

◆ Cigarette smoking
◆ Genetic predisposition
◆ Organic or inorganic dusts and noxious gas exposure
◆ Respiratory tract infection

## *Pathophysiologic changes*

| | |
|---|---|
| Hypersecretion of goblet cells ➡ | **Copious gray, white, or yellow sputum and productive cough** |
| Obstruction of airflow to lower bronchial tree ➡ | **Dyspnea** |
| Hypoxia ➡ | **Tachypnea, cyanosis, and use of accessory muscles for breathing** |
| Narrow, mucus-filled respiratory passages ➡ | **Wheezing and rhonci** |
| Compensatory mechanism to maintain patent airway ➡ | **Prolonged expiratory time** |

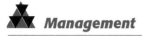

## Management

- Avoidance of air pollutants and smoking cessation — *to decrease irritation*
- Antibiotics — *to treat recurring infections*
- Bronchodilators — *to relieve bronchospasms and facilitate mucociliary clearance*
- Adequate hydration — *to liquefy secretions*
- Chest physiotherapy — *to mobilize secretions*
- Ultrasonic or mechanical nebulizers — *to loosen and mobilize secretions*
- Corticosteroids — *to combat inflammation*
- Diuretics — *to reduce edema*
- Oxygen — *to treat hypoxia*

# Emphysema

◆ Form of chronic obstructive pulmonary disease
◆ Characterized by abnormal, permanent enlargement of acini
  accompanied by destruction of alveolar walls
◆ Airflow limitation caused by lack of elastic recoil in lungs

**THE PATHO PICTURE**

## UNDERSTANDING EMPHYSEMA

In the patient with emphysema, recurrent pulmonary inflammation damages and
eventually destroys the alveolar walls, creating large air spaces. The damaged
alveoli can't recoil normally after expanding; therefore, bronchioles collapse

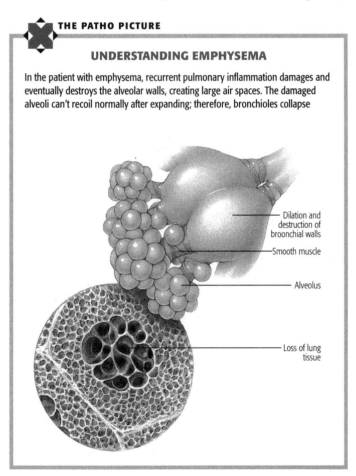

Dilation and destruction of broonchial walls

Smooth muscle

Alveolus

Loss of lung tissue

## *Causes*
◆ Alpha$_1$-antitrypsin (AAT) deficiency
◆ Cigarette smoking

## ▲ *Pathophysiologic changes*

| | |
|---|---|
| Decreased oxygenation ➡ | Tachypnea, dyspnea on exertion |
| Overdistention and overinflation of lungs ➡ | Barrel-shaped chest |
| Accessory muscle use ➡ | Prolonged expiration and grunting |
| Trapped air in alveolar space, alveolar wall destruction ➡ | Decreased breath sounds and tactile fremitus, hyperresonance on chest percussion |
| Chronic hypoxia ➡ | Clubbed fingers and toes |
| Hypoventilation ➡ | Decreased chest expansion |
| Brochiolar collapse ➡ | Crackles and wheezing on inspiration |

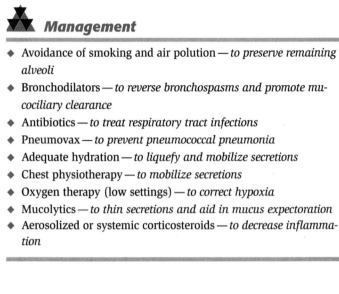 *Management*

◆ Avoidance of smoking and air polution — *to preserve remaining alveoli*
◆ Bronchodilators — *to reverse bronchospasms and promote mucociliary clearance*
◆ Antibiotics — *to treat respiratory tract infections*
◆ Pneumovax — *to prevent pneumococcal pneumonia*
◆ Adequate hydration — *to liquefy and mobilize secretions*
◆ Chest physiotherapy — *to mobilize secretions*
◆ Oxygen therapy (low settings) — *to correct hypoxia*
◆ Mucolytics — *to thin secretions and aid in mucus expectoration*
◆ Aerosolized or systemic corticosteroids — *to decrease inflammation*

# Lung cancer

◆ Development of neoplasm, usually within wall or epithelium of bronchial tree
◆ Most common types: epidermoid (squamous cell) carcinoma, small cell (oat cell) carcinoma, adenocarcinoma, and large cell (anaplastic) carcinoma

**THE PATHO PICTURE**

### HOW LUNG CANCER DEVELOPS

Lung cancer usually begins with the transformation of one epithelial cell within the patient's airway. Although the exact cause of such change remains unclear, some lung cancers originating in the bronchi may be more vulnerable to injuries from carcinogens.

As the tumor grows, it can partially or completely obstruct the airway, resulting in lobar collapse distal to the tumor. Early metastasis may occur to other thoracic structures as well.

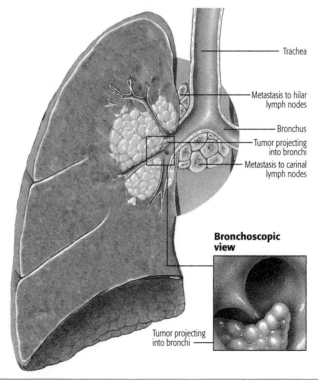

Trachea

Metastasis to hilar lymph nodes

Bronchus

Tumor projecting into bronchi

Metastasis to carinal lymph nodes

**Bronchoscopic view**

Tumor projecting into bronchi

## Causes

◆ Inhalation of carcinogenic and industrial air pollutants
◆ Cigarette smoking
◆ Genetic predisposition

### ▲ *Pathophysiologic changes*

| | |
|---|---|
| Local infiltration of pulmonary membranes and vasculature ➡ | **Cough, hoarseness, wheezing, dyspnea, hemoptysis, chest pain** |
| Hypermetabolic state of tumor cellular proliferation ➡ | **Fever, weight loss, weakness, anorexia** |
| Bronchial obstruction ➡ | **Hemoptysis, atelectasis, pneumonitis, dyspnea** |
| Phrenic nerve compression ➡ | **Shoulder pain, unilateral paralysis of diaphragm** |
| Esophageal compression ➡ | **Dysphagia** |
| Obstruction of vena cava ➡ | **Venous distention; facial, neck and chest edema** |
| Chest wall invasion ➡ | **Piercing chest pain; increasing dyspnea; severe arm pain** |

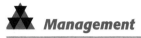 *Management*

◆ Surgical excision of carcinoma; may include partial removal of lung (wedge resection, segmental resection, lobectomy, radical lobectomy) or total removal (pneumonectomy, radical pneumonectomy) — *to remove tumor*

◆ Preoperative radiation therapy — *to reduce tumor bulk and allow for surgical resection*

◆ Radiation therapy (recommended for stage I and stage II lesions; if surgery is contraindicated; for stage III lesions when disease is confined to involved hemithorax and ipsilateral supraclavicular lymph nodes) — *to destroy any cancer cells*

◆ Postsurgical radiation therapy (delayed until 1 month after surgery to allow wound to heal, then directed to part of chest most likely to develop metastasis) — *to destroy any remaining cancer cells*

◆ Chemotherapy — *to induce regression of tumor or prevent metastasis*

◆ Laser therapy (through bronchoscope) — *to destroy local tumors*

# Pneumonia

◆ Acute infection of lung parenchyma that impairs gas exchange
◆ Classified by etiology, location, or type

### THE PATHO PICTURE

## UNDERSTANDING PNEUMONIA

In bacterial pneumonia, an infection triggers alveolar inflammation and edema. This produces an area of low ventilation with normal perfusion. Capillaries become engorged with blood, causing stasis. As the alveocapillary membrane breaks down, alveoli fill with blood and exudates, resulting in atelectasis.

In viral pneumonia, the virus attacks bronchial epithelial cells, causing inflammation and desquamation. The virus also invades mucus glands and goblet cells, spreading to the alveoli, which fill with blood and fluid.

**Lobar pneumonia**

**Bronchopneumonia**

Trachea

Scattered areas of consolidation

Bronchus

Horizontal fissure

Oblique fissure

Oblique fissure

Alveolus

Terminal bronchus

Consolidation in one lobe

## *Causes*

◆ Bacterial or viral infection
◆ Aspiration

## *Risk factors*

◆ Chronic illness and debilitation
◆ Cancer
◆ Abdominal and thoracic surgery
◆ Atelectasis
◆ Chronic respiratory disease
◆ Smoking
◆ Malnutrition

## ◢ *Pathophysiologic changes*

| | |
|---|---|
| Infectious process ➡ | High temperature, pleuritic pain, chills, malaise, tachypnea |
| Pulmonary congestion ➡ | Cough with purulent, yellow or bloody sputum |
| Decreased oxygenation ➡ | Dyspnea |
| Pulmonary congestion ➡ | Crackles, decreased breath sounds |

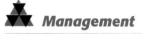 *Management*

- ◆ Antibiotics — *to treat infection*
- ◆ Adequate fluids — *to maintain hydration*
- ◆ Humidified oxygen — *to liquefy secretions*
- ◆ Antitussives — *to promote expectoration*
- ◆ Analgesics — *to relieve pain*
- ◆ Bronchodilators — *to improve oxygenation*
- ◆ High-calorie, high-protein diet — *to maintain nutrition status*
- ◆ Mechanical ventilation (positive end-expiratory pressure) — *for respiratory failure*
- ◆ Drainage of parapneumonic pleural effusion or lung abscess — *to improve lung reexpansion*

# Pneumothorax

◆ Accumulation of air in pleural cavity that leads to partial or complete lung collapse

◆ Most common types: open, closed, and tension

◆ Tension pneumothorax (life-threatening condition that produces most severe symptoms) may result from impeded venous return to heart

◆ Spontaneous pneumothorax (type of closed pneumothorax) is common among older patients with chronic pulmonary disease

**✕ THE PATHO PICTURE**

## UNDERSTANDING PNEUMOTHORAX

### Closed pneumothorax

Closed pneumothorax occurs when air enters the pleural space from within the lung, causing increased pleural pressure, which prevents lung expansion during normal inspiration. This results in a collapsed lung with hypoxia and decreased total lung capacity, vital capacity, and lung compliance.

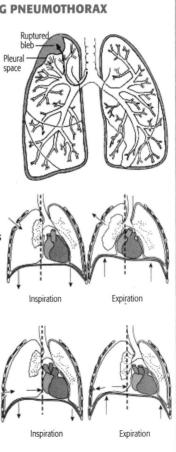

Ruptured bleb

Pleural space

### Open pneumothorax

Open pneumothorax results when atmospheric air flows directly into the pleural cavity on inspiration. As air pressure in the pleural cavity becomes positive, the lung collapses on the affected side during expiration, resulting in decreased total lung capacity, vital capacity, and lung compliance.

Inspiration          Expiration

### Tension pneumothorax

Tension pneumothorax results when air in the pleural space is under higher pressure than air in the adjacent lung. Air enters into the pleural space on inspiration, but cannot escape as the rupture site closes on expiration. Increasing air pressure pushes against the recoiled lung, causing compression atelectasis and displacement of the heart and great vessels.

Inspiration          Expiration

## *Causes*

◆ Open pneumothorax: penetrating chest injury, insertion of central venous catheter, chest surgery, transbronchial biopsy, thoracentesis, closed pleural biopsy
◆ Closed pneumothorax: blunt chest trauma, air leakage from ruptured blebs, rupture resulting from barotrauma, tubercular or cancerous lesions, interstitial lung disease
◆ Tension pneumothorax: penetrating chest wound treated with air-tight dressing, fractured ribs, mechanical ventilation, high-level positive end-expiratory pressure, chest tube occlusion or malfunction

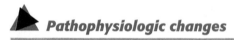 *Pathophysiologic changes*

**OPEN OR CLOSED PNEUMOTHORAX**

| | |
|---|---|
| Lung collapse ➡ | Sudden, sharp pain; asymmetrical chest wall movement; respiratory distress; decreased local fremitus; absent breath sounds (on affected side) |
| Hypoxia ➡ | Shortness of breath, cyanosis, tachycardia |
| Decreased lung expansion ➡ | Chest rigidity (on affected side) |
| Leakage of air into tissues ➡ | Crackling beneath skin on palpation (subcutaneous emphysema) |

**TENSION PNEUMOTHORAX**

| | |
|---|---|
| Decreased cardiac output ➡ | Hypotension; compensatory tachycardia; pallor; weak, rapid pulse |
| Hypoxia ➡ | Tachypnea, anxiety |
| Increased tension ➡ | Mediastinal shift |
| Mediastinal shift ➡ | Tracheal deviation (to opposite side) |

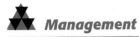 *Management*

**CLOSED PNEUMOTHORAX**

*With less than 30% of lung collapse:*

◆ Bed rest — *to conserve energy and reduce oxygenation demands*

◆ Careful monitoring of respiratory rate, blood pressure, and pulse — *for early detection of physiologic compromise*

◆ Oxygen therapy — *to enhance oxygenation and improve hypoxia*

◆ Aspiration of air with large-bore needle attached to syringe — *to restore negative pressure within pleural space*

*With more than 30% of lung collapse:*

◆ Thoracostomy tube (connected to underwater-seal and low-pressure suction) — *to reexpand lung by restoring negative intrapleural pressure*

◆ Thoracotomy and pleurectomy (may be performed for recurrent spontaneous pneumothorax) — *to adhere lung to parietal pleura*

**OPEN PNEUMOTHORAX**

◆ Chest tube drainage — *to reexpand lung*

◆ Surgery — *to repair lung*

**TENSION PNEUMOTHORAX**

◆ Immediate insertion of large-bore needle into pleural space through second intercostal space — *to reexpand lung*

◆ Insertion of thoracostomy tube — *to rexpand lung*

◆ Analgesics — *to promote comfort and encourage deep breathing and coughing*

# Pulmonary edema

♦ Accumulation of fluid in extravascular spaces of lung
♦ Common complication of cardiovascular disorders
♦ May be chronic or acute

**THE PATHO PICTURE**

### UNDERSTANDING PULMONARY EDEMA

In pulmonary edema, diminished function of the left ventricle causes blood to back up into pulmonary veins and capillaries. The increasing capillary hydrostatic pressure pushes fluid into the interstitial spaces and alveoli. These illustrations show a normal alveolus and an alveolus affected by pulmonary edema.

**Normal alveolus**

Bronchiole

Arterial blood rich with oxygen

Alveolus

Pulmonary artery with mixed venous blood

**Alveolus in pulmonary edema**

Bronchiole

Alveolus

Arterial blood lacking oxygen

Pulmonary artery with mixed venous blood

Interstitial congestion

## *Causes*

- ◆ Left-sided heart failure
- ◆ Diastolic dysfunction
- ◆ Valvular heart disease
- ◆ Arrhythmias
- ◆ Fluid overload
- ◆ Acute myocardial ischemia and infarction
- ◆ Barbiturate or opiate poisoning
- ◆ Inhalation of irritating gases
- ◆ Left atrial myxoma
- ◆ Pneumonia

## ▲ *Pathophysiologic changes*

**EARLY STAGES**

Hypoxia ➡ Dyspnea on exertion, mild tachypnea, cough, tachycardia

Decreased ability of diaphragm to expand ➡ Orthopnea

Increased pulmonary pressures ➡ Increased blood pressure

Fluid-filled lungs ➡ Dependent crackles

Decreased cardiac output and increased pulmonary vascular resistance ➡ Neck vein distention

**LATER STAGES**

Hypoxia ➡ Labored, rapid respiration; increased tachycardia; cyanosis; arrhythmias

Fluid-filled lungs ➡ More diffuse crackles, cough (producing frothy, bloody sputum)

Peripheral vasoconstriction ➡ Cold, clammy skin

Decreased cardiac output, shock ➡ Diaphoresis, decreased blood pressure, thready pulse

# ▲▲▲ *Management*

- ◆ High concentrations of oxygen (administered by nasal cannula) — *to enhance gas exchange and improve oxygenation*
- ◆ Assisted ventilation — *to improve oxygen delivery to tissues and promote acid-base balance*
- ◆ Diuretics (furosemide, bumetanide) — *to increase urination, which helps mobilize extravascular fluid*
- ◆ Positive inotropic agents (digoxin, inamrinone) — *to enhance contractility in myocardial dysfunction*
- ◆ Pressor agents — *to enhance contractility and promote vasoconstriction in peripheral vessels*
- ◆ Antiarrhythmics — *for arrhythmias related to decreased cardiac output*
- ◆ Arterial vasodilators (nitroprusside) — *to decrease peripheral vascular resistance, preload, and afterload*
- ◆ Morphine — *to reduce anxiety and dyspnea and to dilate systemic venous bed (thereby promoting blood flow from pulmonary circulation to periphery)*

# Pulmonary embolism

◆ Obstruction of pulmonary arterial bed by dislodged thrombus, heart valve growth, or foreign substance
◆ Most common pulmonary complication in hospitalized patients; massive embolism may be fatal

## HOW IT HAPPENS

Blood clot forms in the deep venous system.

Clot dislodges and travels through systemic venous system, right chambers of heart, and into pulmonary circulation.

Clot lodges in branch of circulatory system.

Blood flow distal to obstruction is blocked.

Embolus prevents alveoli from producing enough surfactant to maintain alveolar integrity; alveoli collapse and atelectasis develops.

Large clot can cause tissue death.

## *Causes*

◆ Deep vein thrombosis
◆ Pelvic, renal, and hepatic vein thrombosis
◆ Right heart thrombus
◆ Upper extremity thrombosis
◆ Atrial fibrillation
◆ Valvular heart disease

## *Risk factors*

◆ Long-term immobility
◆ Recent surgery
◆ Obesity
◆ High-estrogen oral contraceptive use
◆ Long car or plane trips

## ▲ *Pathophysiologic changes*

| | |
|---|---|
| Hypoxemia ➧ | Tachycardia; dyspnea, signs of circulatory collapse (weak, thready pulse; hypotension), respiratory alkalosis |
| Inflammatory process ➧ | Low-grade fever |
| Vasoconstriction and right-sided heart failure ➧ | Hemoptysis, cyanosis, syncope, and distended neck veins (occur with massive embolism) |

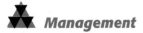 *Management*

- Oygen therapy — *to treat hypoxemia*
- Anticoagulation (with heparin) — *to inhibit new thrombus formation*
- Fibrinolytic therapy — *to enhance fibrinolysis of pulmonary emboli and remaining thrombi*
- Vasopressors — *to treat hypotension*
- Antibiotics — *to treat septic emboli*
- Vena caval ligation, plication, or insertion of device (umbrella filter) — *to filter blood returning to heart and lungs*

# Pulmonary hypertension

◆ Increase in pulmonary artery pressure (PAP) above normal (mean PAP of 25 mm Hg or more) that occurs for reasons other than aging or altitude
◆ May be classified as primary (idiopathic) or secondary
  – Primary characterized by increased PAP and increased pulmonary vascular resistance (with no obvious cause); most common in women aged 20 to 40
  – Secondary results from existing cardiac or pulmonary disease (or both)

**✦ THE PATHO PICTURE**

### UNDERSTANDING PULMONARY HYPERTENSION

Smooth muscle in the pulmonary artery wall hypertrophies for no reason, narrowing the small pulmonary artery (arterioles) or obliterating it completely. Fibrous lesions also form around the vessels, impairing distensibility and increasing vascular resistance. Increased pressures generated in the lungs are transmitted to the right ventricle, which supplies the pulmonary artery. Eventually, the right ventricle fails.

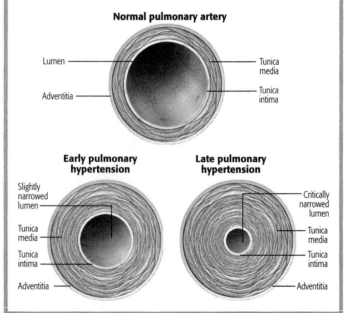

**Normal pulmonary artery**

Lumen — Tunica media
Adventitia — Tunica intima

**Early pulmonary hypertension**

Slightly narrowed lumen
Tunica media
Tunica intima
Adventitia

**Late pulmonary hypertension**

Critically narrowed lumen
Tunica media
Tunica intima
Adventitia

## Causes

◆ Primary pulmonary hypertension: possibly hereditary factors or altered immune mechanisms
◆ Secondary pulmonary hypertension: chronic obstructive pulmonary disease, diffuse interstitial pneumonia, malignant metastases, scleroderma, obesity, pulmonary embolism, vasculitis, rheumatic valvular disease, mitral stenosis

## ◤ Pathophysiologic changes

| | |
|---|---|
| Left-sided heart failure ▶ | Increasing dyspnea on exertion; difficulty breathing; shortness of breath; restlessness, agitation, decreased level of consciousness, confusion, memory loss |
| Diminished tissue oxygenation ▶ | Fatigue and weakness; syncope |
| Buildup of lactic acid in tissues ▶ | Pain with breathing |
| Right ventricular failure ▶ | Ascites, neck vein distention, peripheral edema |
| Hypoventilation ▶ | Decreased diaphragmatic excursion and respiration |
| Fluid accumulation in lungs ▶ | Possible displacement of point of maximal impulse beyond midclavicular line; decreased breath sounds; loud, tubular breath sounds |
| Altered cardiac output ▶ | Easily palpable right ventricular lift; systolic ejection murmur; split S2, S3, and S4 |

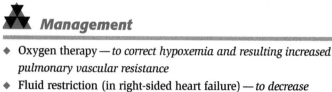

## *Management*

◆ Oxygen therapy — *to correct hypoxemia and resulting increased pulmonary vascular resistance*
◆ Fluid restriction (in right-sided heart failure) — *to decrease heart's workload*
◆ Digoxin — *to increase cardiac output*
◆ Diuretics — *to decrease intravascular volume and extravascular fluid accumulation*
◆ Vasodilators — *to reduce myocardial workload and oxygen consumption*
◆ Calcium channel blockers — *to reduce myocardial workload and oxygen consumption*
◆ Bronchodilators — *to relax smooth muscles and increase airway patency*
◆ Beta-adrenergic blockers — *to improve oxygenation*
◆ Treatment of underlying cause — *to correct pulmonary edema*
◆ Heart-lung transplant — *to treat severe cases*

# Severe acute respiratory syndrome (SARS)

◆ Life-threatening viral infection
◆ Incubation period estimated to range from 2 to 7 days (average 3 to 5 days)
◆ Not highly contagious when protective measures are used

**THE PATHO PICTURE**

## UNDERSTANDING SARS

Although the exact origin of SARS is unknown, close contact with civet cats may have transmitted a mutated form of the coronavirus to humans. Viral infection of a human host cell could occur as follows:

The SARS virion (A) attaches to receptors on the host-cell membrane and releases enzymes (called absorption) (B) that weaken the membrane and enable the SARS virion to penetrate the cell. The SARS virion removes the protein coat that protects its genetic material (C), replicates (D), and matures, and then escapes from the cell by budding from the plasma membrane (E). The infection then can spread to other host cells.

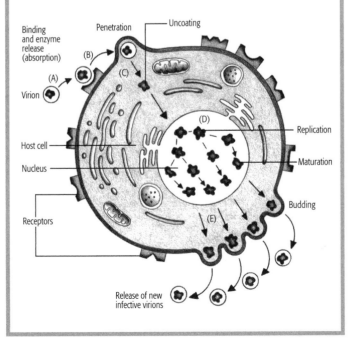

## Cause

♦ Transmission of new type of coronavirus known as *SARS-associated coronavirus* (SARS-CoV)

## Risk factors

♦ Close contact with infected person
♦ Contact with aerosolized (exhaled) droplets and bodily secretions from infected person
♦ Travel to endemic areas

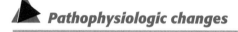 **Pathophysiologic changes**

Infectious process 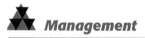     Nonproductive cough, rash, high fever, headache, general discomfort and body aches, pneumonia

Decreased oxygenation ➡     Shortness of breath, respiratory distress (in later stages)

## Management

♦ Isolation (for hospitalized patients) — *to prevent spread of disease*
♦ Strict respiratory and mucosal barrier precautions — *to prevent spread of disease*
♦ Quarantine (of exposed people) — *to prevent spread of disease*
♦ Mechanical ventilation (for severe cases) — *to treat respiratory failure*
♦ Diet (as tolerated) — *to provide adequate nutrition*
♦ Global surveillance and reporting of suspected cases to national health authorities — *to monitor spread of disease*
♦ Antivirals — *to treat viral infection*
♦ Combination of steroids and antimicrobials — *to treat inflammation and infection*

# Tuberculosis

◆ Lung infection characterized by pulmonary infiltrates and formation of granulomas with caseation, fibrosis, and cavitation
◆ May be acute or chronic
◆ Prognosis excellent with proper treatment and compliance

**THE PATHO PICTURE**

**UNDERSTANDING TUBERCULOSIS INVASION**

After infected droplets are inhaled, they are deposited in the lungs. Leukocytes surround the droplets, leading to inflammation. As part of the inflammatory response, some mycobacteria enter the lymphatic circulation via the lymph nc

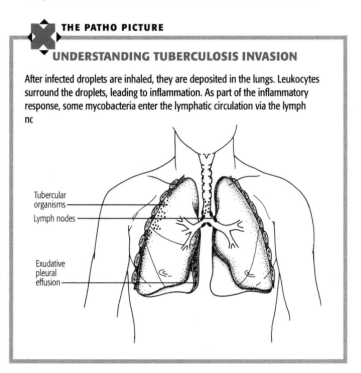

Tubercular organisms

Lymph nodes

Exudative pleural effusion

## *Causes*

◆ Exposure to *Mycobacterium tuberculosis*
◆ Sometimes, exposure to other strains of mycobacteria

## *Risk factors*

◆ Close contact with newly diagnosed patient
◆ History of prior tuberculosis exposure
◆ Multiple sexual partners
◆ Recent emigration (from Africa, Asia, Mexico, South America)
◆ Gastrectomy
◆ History of silicosis, diabetes, malnutrition, cancer, Hodgkin's disease, leukemia
◆ Drug or alcohol abuse
◆ Residence in nursing home, mental health facility, prison
◆ Immunosuppression, corticosteroid use
◆ Homelessness

## *Pathophysiologic changes*

| Inflammatory and immune process ➤ | Fever and night sweats; malaise, weight loss; adenopathy; productive cough (lasting longer than 3 weeks); hemoptysis, pleuritic chest pain |
| --- | --- |

## *Management*

◆ Antitubercular therapy (for at least 6 months with daily oral doses) — *to treat infection*
◆ Resumption of normal activities while taking medication (after 2 to 4 weeks, when disease is no longer infectious) — *to promote independence*
◆ Well-balanced, high-calorie diet — *to maintain or improve nutritional status*

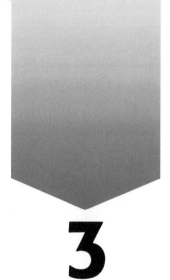

# 3

# Neurologic disorders

# PATHOPHYSIOLOGIC CONCEPTS

## *Altered arousal*

◆ Can result from:
  – direct destruction of reticular activating system (RAS) and its pathways
  – destruction of entire brain stem, either directly by invasion or indirectly by impairment of its blood supply
  – compression of RAS by disease, from either direct pressure or compression as structures expand or herniate
  – structural, metabolic, or psychogenic disturbances

### STAGES OF ALTERED AROUSAL

◆ Begins with interruption or disruption in diencephalon
◆ Manifestations based on six states of altered consciousness: confusion, disorientation, lethargy, obtundation, stupor, and coma
◆ Cause of alteration determined by evaluating neurologic function with regard to:
  – level of consciousness
  – breathing pattern
  – pupillary changes
  – eye movement and reflex responses
  – motor responses

## *Altered homeostasis*

◆ Failure in brain's normal autoregulatory mechanisms
◆ Can result in increased intracranial pressure (ICP) and cerebral edema

### INCREASED ICP

◆ Pressure exerted by brain tissue, cerebrospinal fluid (CSF), and cerebral blood (intracranial components) against skull
◆ Change in volume of intracranial contents triggers reciprocal change in one or more intracranial components to maintain consistent pressure
◆ Compensatory mechanisms attempt to maintain homeostasis and lower ICP
◆ ICP continues to rise when compensatory mechanisms are overwhelmed and no longer effective

## WHEN ICP RISES

The brain compensates for increases in intracranial pressure by:
◆ limiting blood flow to the head
◆ displacing CSF into the spinal canal
◆ increasing absorption or decreasing production of CSF (withdrawing water from brain tissue and excreting it through the kidneys).

When compensatory mechanisms become overworked, small changes in volume can lead to large changes in pressure.

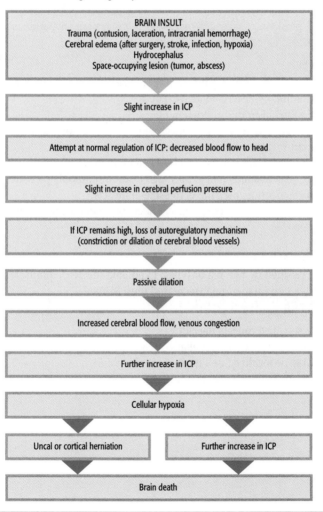

BRAIN INSULT
Trauma (contusion, laceration, intracranial hemorrhage)
Cerebral edema (after surgery, stroke, infection, hypoxia)
Hydrocephalus
Space-occupying lesion (tumor, abscess)

Slight increase in ICP

Attempt at normal regulation of ICP: decreased blood flow to head

Slight increase in cerebral perfusion pressure

If ICP remains high, loss of autoregulatory mechanism
(constriction or dilation of cerebral blood vessels)

Passive dilation

Increased cerebral blood flow, venous congestion

Further increase in ICP

Cellular hypoxia

Uncal or cortical herniation

Further increase in ICP

Brain death

**CEREBRAL EDEMA**

♦ Characterized as increase in fluid content of brain tissue that leads to increase in intracellular or extracellular fluid volume
♦ May result from initial injury to brain tissue
♦ May develop in response to cerebral ischemia, hypoxia, and hypercapnia

## Altered movement

♦ Certain neurotransmitters (such as dopamine) play a role
♦ Typically characterized by excessive movement (hyperkinesia) or decreased movement (hypokinesia)

**PARESIS**

♦ Partial loss of motor function (paralysis) and muscle power
♦ Commonly described as weakness
♦ Can result from dysfunction of:
  – upper motor neurons (in cerebral cortex, subcortical white matter, internal capsule, brain stem, or spinal cord)
  – lower motor neurons (in brain stem motor nuclei and anterior horn of spinal cord); may also result from problems with their axons as they travel to skeletal muscle
  – motor units affecting muscle fibers or neuromuscular junction

## Altered muscle tone

♦ Classified by two major types: hypotonia (decreased muscle tone) and hypertonia (increased muscle tone)

**HYPOTONIA**

♦ Also called muscle flaccidity
♦ Typically reflects cerebellar damage
♦ May be localized to a limb or muscle group
♦ May be generalized, affecting entire body

### *HYPERTONIA*

◆ Increased resistance to passive movement
◆ Four types of hypertonia:
  – spasticity (hyperexcitability of stretch reflexes caused by damage to lateral corticospinal tract and to motor, premotor, and supplementary motor areas)
  – paratonia (variance in resistance to passive movement in direct proportion to force applied)
  – dystonia (sustained, involuntary twisting movements resulting from slow muscle contraction)
  – rigidity (constant, involuntary muscle contraction resulting in resistance during flexion and extension)

## *Impaired cognition*

◆ Alteration resulting from:
  – direct destruction by ischemia and hypoxia
  – indirect destruction by compression
  – effects of toxins and chemicals
◆ May manifest as:
  – agnosia (defect in ability to recognize form or nature of objects)
  – aphasia (loss of ability to comprehend or produce language)
  – dysphasia (impaired ability to comprehend or use symbols in verbal or written language, or to produce language)

### *DEMENTIA*

◆ Loss of more than one intellectual or cognitive function, which interferes with ability to function in daily life
◆ May cause problems with orientation, general knowledge and information, vigilance, recent or remote memory, concept formulation, abstraction, reasoning, or language use
◆ Underlying mechanism: defect in neuronal circuitry of brain
◆ Classified according to three major types: amnestic, intentional, and cognitive

# DISORDERS

## Alzheimer's disease

◆ Degenerative disorder of cerebral cortex (especially frontal lobe and hippocampus) that is considered primary progressive form of dementia
◆ Accounts for more than half of all cases of dementia
◆ Carries poor prognosis

**THE PATHO PICTURE**

### ABNORMAL CELLULAR STRUCTURES IN ALZHEIMER'S DISEASE

How and why neurons die in Alzheimer's disease is largely unknown. The brain tissue of patients with Alzheimer's disease exhibits three distinct and characteristic features: granulovacuolar degeneration, neurofibrillary tangles, and amyloid plaques.

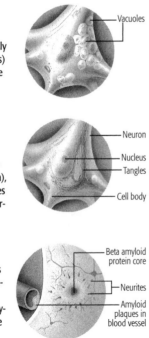

#### Granulovacuolar degeneration
This type of degeneration occurs inside the neurons of the hippocampus. An abnormally high number of fluid-filled spaces (vacuoles) enlarge the cell's body, possibly causing the cell to die.

Vacuoles

#### Neurofibrillary tangles
These are bundles of filaments inside the neuron that abnormally twist around one another. They are found in the brain areas associated with memory and learning (hippocampus), fear and aggression (amygdala), and thinking (cerebral cortex). These tangles may play a role in the memory loss and personality changes that commonly occur in Alzheimer's disease.

Neuron
Nucleus
Tangles
Cell body

#### Amyloid plaques
Also called senile plaques, amyloid plaques are found outside neurons in the extracellular space of the cerebral cortex and hippocampus. They contain a core of beta amyloid protein surrounded by abnormal nerve endings (neurites).

Beta amyloid protein core
Neurites
Amyloid plaques in blood vessel

## Causes

◆ Exact cause unknown
◆ Neurochemical factors: deficiencies in neurotransmitters acetylcholine, serotonin, somatostatin, and norepinephrine
◆ Environmental factors: repeated head trauma; exposure to aluminum or manganese

## Risk factors

◆ Family history of Alzheimer's disease
◆ Presence of Down syndrome

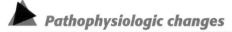 **Pathophysiologic changes**

| | |
|---|---|
| Neurotransmitter metabolism defects ➡ | **Initial stage:** Gradual loss of recent and remote memory; disorientation (time, date); flattening of affect and personality |
| Neurotransmitter metabolism deficits or structural loss of brain tissue ➡ | **Progressive stages:** Impaired cognition; inability to concentrate; difficulty with abstraction and judgment; inability to perform activities of daily living; restlessness and agitation; personality changes; nocturnal awakening and wandering; severe deterioration in memory, language, and motor function; loss of coordination; inability to write or speak; loss of eye contact; acute confusion, agitation, compulsive behavior, fearfulness; disorientation and emotional lability; urinary and fecal incontinence |

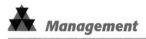

## Management

- ◆ Cholinesterase inhibition therapy — *to help improve memory deficits*
- ◆ N-methyl-D-aspartate (NMDA) receptor antagonist therapy — *to improve memory and learning of patients with moderate to severe Alzheimer's disease*
- ◆ Antidepressants — *to improve mood and reduce irritability*
- ◆ Antipsychotics — *to treat hallucinations, delusions, aggression, hostility, uncooperativeness*
- ◆ Antioxidant therapy (vitamin E therapy under current study) — *to possibly delay disease effects*
- ◆ Anxiolytics — *for anxiety, restlessness, verbally disruptive behavior, resistance*
- ◆ Behavioral interventions (simplifying environment, tasks, routines) — *to prevent agitation*
- ◆ Effective communication strategies — *to ensure continued communication between patient and family*
- ◆ Teaching aids, social service and community references — *for educating care-givers and for legal and financial advice and support*

# Amyotrophic lateral sclerosis (ALS)

◆ Chronic, progressively debilitating disease, commonly called
  Lou Gehrig's disease
◆ Most common form of motor neuron disease causing muscular
  atrophy
◆ Onset usually occurs between ages 40 and 60
◆ Affects men twice as often as women

---

### HOW IT HAPPENS

ALS progressively destroys upper and lower motor neurons (including anterior
horn cells of the spinal cord, upper motor neurons of the cerebral cortex, and
motor nuclei of the brain stem).

> May begin when glutamate (primary excitatory neurotransmitter of CNS) accumulates
> to toxic levels at synapses.

> Affected motor units are no longer innervated; progressive degeneration of axons
> causes loss of myelin.

> Nonfunctional scar tissue replaces normal neuronal tissue; denervation leads to muscle
> fiber atrophy and motor neuron degeneration.

---

## *Causes*

◆ Exact cause unknown; 5% to 10% of cases have genetic component
◆ Possible contributing mechanisms:
  – slow-acting virus
  – nutritional deficiency related to disturbance in enzyme metabolism
  – unknown mechanism that causes buildup of excess gluta-
  mine in cerebrospinal fluid
  – autoimmune diorder

# ▲ *Pathophysiologic changes*

| Degeneration of upper and lower motor neurons ➡ | Fasciculations accompanied by spasticity, atrophy, hyperreflexia and weakness (especially in muscles of forearms and hands), muscle atrophy |

| Degeneration of cranial nerves V, IX, X, and XII ➡ | Impaired speech, difficulty chewing and swallowing, choking, and excessive drooling |

| Brain stem involvement ➡ | **Difficulty breathing** |

| Progressive bulbar palsy ➡ | **Emotional lability** |

# ▲ *Management*

◆ Supportive medical intervention (ALS has no cure):
  – diazepam, dantrolene, or baclofen — *to decrease spasticity*
  – quinidine — *to relieve painful muscle cramps*
  – thyrotropin-releasing hormone — *to temporarily improve motor function*
  – riluzole — *to modulate glutamate activity and slow disease progression*
◆ Respiratory, speech, and physical therapy — *to maintain as much function as possible*
◆ Psychological support — *to assist with coping*
◆ Rehabilitation program — *to maintain independence as long as possible*
◆ Referral to hospice or local ALS support group — *as supportive care for patient and family*

# Intracranial aneurysm

◆ Weakness in wall of cerebral artery; causes localized dilation
◆ Usually arises at arterial junction in Circle of Willis
◆ Rupture (typically abrupt, without warning) is common, resulting in subarachnoid hemorrhage
◆ Severity of rupture is graded according to signs and symptoms
◆ Incidence is slightly higher in women than in men, especially those in late 40s or early to mid-50s

**THE PATHO PICTURE**

**HOW A CEREBRAL ANEURYSM DEVELOPS**

In an intracranial (cerebral) aneurysm, weakness in the wall of a cerebral artery causes localized dilation. Blood flow exerts pressure against the wall, stretching it like a balloon and making it likely to rupture. Cerebral aneurysms usually arise at the arterial bifurcation in the Circle of Willis and its branches. This illustration shows the most common sites around this circle.

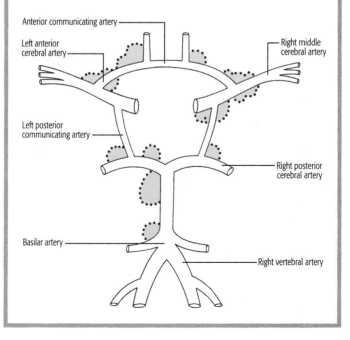

Anterior communicating artery

Left anterior cerebral artery

Right middle cerebral artery

Left posterior communicating artery

Right posterior cerebral artery

Basilar artery

Right vertebral artery

## *Causes*

- ◆ Congenital defect
- ◆ Degenerative process
- ◆ Combination of congenital defect and degenerative process
- ◆ Traumatic injury

## ▲ *Pathophysiologic changes*

**PREMONITORY STAGE**

Oozing of blood into subarachnoid space ➡ | Headache, intermittent nausea, vomiting; nuchal rigidity; stiff back and legs

**RUPTURE STAGE**

Increased pressure from bleeding into enclosed space ➡ | Sudden, severe headache; nausea and projectile vomiting; altered level of consciousness, including deep coma (depends on severity of rupture and location of bleeding)

Bleeding into meninges ➡ | Meningeal irritation
– Nuchal rigidity
– Back and leg pain
– Fever
– Restlessness, irritability
– Occasional seizures, photophobia, blurred vision

Bleeding into brain tissues ➡ | Hemiparesis, hemisensory defects, dysphagia, and visual defects

Compression on oculomotor nerve (if aneurysm is near internal carotid artery) ➡ | Diplopia, ptosis, dilated pupil, inability to rotate eye

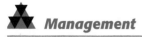 *Management*

- Bed rest in quiet, darkened room with minimal stimulation — *to help reduce risk of rupture*
- Avoidance of coffee, other stimulants, and aspirin — *to reduce risk of blood pressure elevation*
- Codeine or another analgesic — *to promote rest and minimize risk of pressure changes*
- Hydralazine or other antihypertensive agent — *to help reduce risk of rupture*
- Phenobarbital or other sedative — *to prevent agitation leading to hypertension*
- Endotracheal intubation (if necessary) — *to provide adequate airway*
- Surgery (clipping, ligation, or wrapping before or after rupture; endovascular repair) — *to repair aneurysm*
- Calcium channel blockers — *to decrease spasm and subsequent rebleeding*
- Corticosteroids — *to manage headache in subarachnoid hemorrhage*
- Phenytoin or other anticonvulsant — *to prevent or treat seizures secondary to pressure and tissue irritation from bleeding*
- Aminocaproic acid — *to minimize risk of rebleeding by delaying blood clot lysis*

# Lyme disease

◆ Multisystemic disorder caused by *Borrelia burgdorferi* (spirochete transmitted through tick bite)
◆ Primarily occurs in areas inhabited by small deer tick *(Ixodes dammini)*
◆ Typically manifests in three stages:
  – Early localized stage (distinctive red rash accompanied by flulike symptoms)
  – Early disseminated stage (neurologic and cardiac abnormalities)
  – Late stage (arthritis, chronic neurologic problems)

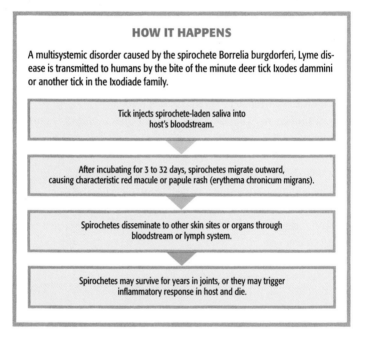

**HOW IT HAPPENS**

A multisystemic disorder caused by the spirochete Borrelia burgdorferi, Lyme disease is transmitted to humans by the bite of the minute deer tick Ixodes dammini or another tick in the Ixodiade family.

Tick injects spirochete-laden saliva into host's bloodstream.

After incubating for 3 to 32 days, spirochetes migrate outward, causing characteristic red macule or papule rash (erythema chronicum migrans).

Spirochetes disseminate to other skin sites or organs through bloodstream or lymph system.

Spirochetes may survive for years in joints, or they may trigger inflammatory response in host and die.

## Causes

◆ Infestation of spirochete *Borrelia burgdorferi* resulting from tick bite (injects spirochete-laden saliva into bloodstream or deposits fecal matter on skin)

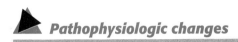

# Pathophysiologic changes

### EARLY LOCALIZED STAGE

Local infection of *B. burgdorferi* spirochete ➡

Distinctive red rash (erythema chronicum migrans) that appears as target or bull's eye (commonly at site of tick bite), flulike symptoms (fever, chills, myalgias, headache, malaise), regional lymphadenopathy

### EARLY DISSEMINATED STAGE

Dissemination of spirochetes into bloodstream ➡

Neurologic abnormalities (peripheral and cranial neuropathy), cardiac abnormalities (carditis, conduction disturbances), eye abnormalities (conjunctivitis)

### LATE STAGE

Presence of organisms in synovium ➡

Inflammation, joint swelling, arthritis

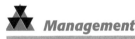

# Management

- ◆ Antibiotics — *to treat infection*
  – Early localized disease: doxycycline or amoxicillin for 3 to 4 weeks, or cefuroxime axetil or erythromycin if patient is allergic to penicillin or tetracycline
  – Late disease: I.V. cefitriaxone or penicillin for 4 or more weeks
- ◆ Anti-inflammatory agents — *to treat arthritis*
- ◆ Close monitoring for ptosis, strabismus, diplopia — *for signs of increased intracranial pressure and cranial nerve involvement*
- ◆ Monitoring of heart rate and rhythm — *to detect arrhythmias*

# Meningitis

- ◆ Inflammation of brain and spinal cord meninges, usually resulting from bacterial infection
- ◆ May involve inflammation of all three meningeal membranes: dura mater, arachnoid, and pia mater
- ◆ Rarely any complications, especially when disease is recognized early and infecting organism responds to treatment
- ◆ Generally good prognosis (poorer for infants and elderly patients)

**THE PATHO PICTURE**

### INFLAMMATION IN MENINGITIS

In meningitis, pathogens trigger an inflammatory response in the brain and spinal cord. Often, inflammation begins in the pia-arachnoid (pia mater and arachnoid space) and progresses to congestion of adjacent tissues, where exudates cause nerve cell destruction and increased intracranial pressure. This results in engorged blood vessels, disrupted blood supply, thrombosis or rupture, and possibly cerebral infarction.

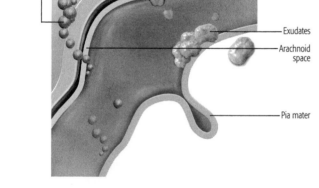

## *Causes*

- Most commonly, as complication of bacterial infection in pneumonia, empyema, osteomyelitis, endocarditis
- Other possible infections: sinusitis, otitis media, encephalitis, brain abscess (from *Neisseria meningitidis, Haemophilus influenzae, Streptococcus pneumoniae,* or *Escherichia coli*)
- Trauma or invasive procedures
- Virus or other organism (aseptic meningitis)
- No causative organism (in some cases)

## *Pathophysiologic changes*

| | |
|---|---|
| Infection and inflammation ➡ | **Fever, chills, and malaise** |
| Increased intracranial pressure (ICP) ➡ | **Headache, vomiting and, papilledema (rarely)** |
| Meningeal irritation ➡ | **Nuchal rigidity; positive Brudzinski's and Kernig's signs; exaggerated and symmetrical deep tendon reflexes; opisthotonos** |
| Irritation of nerves of autonomic nervous system ➡ | **Sinus arrhythmias** |
| Increasing ICP ➡ | **Irritability, delirium, deep stupor, coma** |
| Cranial nerve irritation ➡ | **Photophobia, diplopia, and other vision problems** |

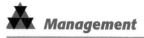

## Management

- I.V. antibiotics (for at least 2 weeks) followed by oral antibiotics — *to treat infection*
- Digoxin — *to control arrhythmias*
- Mannitol — *to decrease cerebral edema*
- Anticonvulsants or sedatives — *to reduce restlessness and prevent or control seizures*
- Aspirin or acetaminophen — *to relieve headache and fever*
- Bed rest — *to prevent increases in ICP*
- Fever reduction — *to prevent hyperthermia and increased metabolic demands that may increase ICP*
- Fluid therapy (cautiously with cerebral edema and increased ICP) — *to maintain fluid balance*
- Prophylactic antibiotics (after ventricular shunting procedures, skull fracture, or penetrating head wounds) — *to prevent infection*
- Droplet precautions (in addition to standard precautions for meningitis caused by *H. influenzae* and *N. meningitidis;* given until 24 hours after start of effective therapy) — *to prevent transmission*

# Migraine headache

◆ Throbbing, vascular headache that usually appears in childhood and often recurs throughout adulthood
◆ May be classified according to presence of aura
  – common migraine, no aura (80% of cases)
  – classic migraine, with aura (20% of cases)
◆ More common in women; strong familial incidence

**THE PATHO PICTURE**

## HOW MIGRAINE HEADACHE DEVELOPS

Migraine headaches are thought to be associated with constriction and dilation of intracranial and extracranial arteries. Neurogenic inflammation can cause local vasoconstriction of innervated cerebral arteries and reduced cerebral blood flow. This causes compensatory vasodilation and biochemical abnormalities, including local leakage of neurokinin through dilated arteries and decreased plasma level of serotonin.

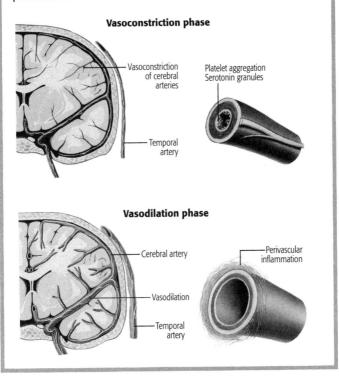

**Vasoconstriction phase**

Vasoconstriction of cerebral arteries

Platelet aggregation
Serotonin granules

Temporal artery

**Vasodilation phase**

Cerebral artery

Perivascular inflammation

Vasodilation

Temporal artery

## *Causes*

- ◆ Exact cause unknown
- ◆ Triggering mechanism may be neuronal dysfunction, possibly of trigeminal nerve pathway
- ◆ Contributing triggering factors include:
  - change in routine (sleep, weather, hormonal)
  - missed meals
  - caffeine intake
  - emotional stress or fatigue
- ◆ environmental stimuli (noise, crowds, bright lights)

## ▲ *Pathophysiologic changes*

| | |
|---|---|
| Neurogenic inflammation, constriction and dilation of cranial arteries ➡ | **Unilateral, pulsating pain** |
| Neurogenic inflammation ➡ | **Prodromal symptoms: scintillating scotoma (appearance of zigzag lines), hemianopia, unilateral paresthesia, or speech disorders** |
| Neurogenic inflammation and autonomic nervous system response ➡ | **Irritability, anorexia, nausea, vomiting, and photophobia** |

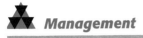 *Management*

- ◆ Abortive medications (5HT1-receptor agonists, dihydroergota-mine, nonsteroidal anti-inflammatory drugs) — *for pain relief (early treatment of symptoms is most effective)*
- ◆ Beta-blockers, clonidine, amitriptyline — *to prevent migraine attacks*
- ◆ Antiemetic drugs — *for nausea and vomiting*
- ◆ Biofeedback and massage — *to relieve or reduce pain*
- ◆ Avoidance of trigger factors — *to prevent migraine attacks*
- ◆ Maintenance of headache diary — *to help determine headache triggers*

# Multiple sclerosis

◆ Chronic disease characterized by progressive demyelination of white matter of brain and spinal cord, with periods of exacerbation and remission

◆ Major cause of chronic disability in young adults (average age of onset is 27)

◆ More common among women (three women for every two men) and in urban populations and upper socioeconomic groups

**THE PATHO PICTURE**

## HOW MYELIN BREAKS DOWN

Myelin speeds electrical impulses to the brain for interpretation. This lipoprotein complex (formed of glial cells or oligodendrocytes) protects the neuron's axon much like the insulation on an electrical wire. Its high electrical resistance and low capacitance allow the myelin to conduct nerve impulses from one node of Ranvier to the next.

Myelin is susceptible to injury (for example, by hypoxemia, toxic chemicals, vascular insufficiencies, or autoimmune responses). The sheath becomes inflamed, and the membrane layers break down into smaller components that become well-circumscribed plaques (filled with microglial elements, macroglia, and lymphocytes). This process is called demyelination.

The damaged myelin sheath can't conduct normally. The partial loss or dispersion of the action potential causes neurologic dysfunction.

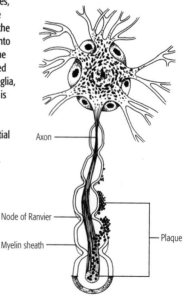

**Abnormal neuron**

Axon

Node of Ranvier

Myelin sheath

Plaque

## *Causes*

◆ Exact cause unknown
◆ Possibly caused by slow-acting or latent viral infection that triggers autoimmune response or by environmental or genetic factors
◆ Conditions that may precede onset or exacerbation: emotional stress, fatigue (physical or emotional), pregnancy, acute respiratory infections

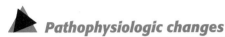

### *Pathophysiologic changes*

| | |
|---|---|
| Conduction deficits, impaired impulse transmission along nerve fiber ➡ | Initial symptoms:<br>– vision problems<br>– sensory impairment (burning, paresthesia, and electrical sensations)<br>– fatigue |
| Cranial nerve dysfunction, conduction defects in optic - nerve ➡ | Ocular disturbances (optic neuritis, diplopia, ophthalmoplegia, blurred vision, and nystagmus) |
| Impaired motor reflex ➡ | Muscle dysfunction (weakness; paralysis ranging from monoplegia to quadriplegia; spasticity; hyperreflexia; intention tremor; gait ataxia) |
| Impaired sphincter innervation ➡ | Urinary disturbances (incontinence, frequency, urgency, frequent infections); bowel disturbances (involuntary evacuation or constipation) |
| Impaired impulse transmission to cranial nerves and sensory cortex) ➡ | Speech problems (poorly articulated or scanning speech; dysphagia) |

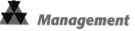 *Management*

- I.V. methylprednisolone followed by oral therapy (azathioprine or methotrexate, cytoxin may be used) — *to reduce edema of myelin sheath (speeds recovery from acute attacks)*
- Immunotherapy (interferon, glatiramer) — *to reduce frequency and severity of relapses and possibly slow central nervous system damage*
- Stretching and range-of-motion exercises (coupled with correct positioning) — *to relieve spasticity resulting from opposing muscle groups relaxing and contracting at same time*
- Baclofen, tizanidine — *to treat spasticity*
- Botulinum toxin injections, intrathecal injections, nerve blocks, or surgery — *for severe spasticity*
- Frequent rest, aerobic exercise, and cooling techniques (air conditioning, breezes, water sprays) — *to help minimize fatigue*
- Amantidine (Symmetrel), pemoline (Cylert), methylphenidate (Ritalin), antidepressants — *to help manage fatigue*
- Cranberry juice, insertion of indwelling catheter and suprapubic tubes, intermittent self-catheterization, postvoid catheterization, anticholinergic drugs — *to help manage bladder control*
- Increased fiber intake, use of bulking agents, bowel-training strategies (daily suppositories and rectal stimulation) — *to help manage bowel problems*
- Low-dose tricyclic antidepressants, phenytoin, or carbamazepine — *to manage sensory symptoms (pain, numbness, burning, and tingling)*
- Adaptive devices and physical therapy — *to assist with motor dysfunction*
- Beta-adrenergic blockers, sedatives, or diuretics — *to alleviate tremor*
- Speech therapy — *to treat dysarthria*
- Antihistamines, vision therapy — *to minimize vertigo*

# Myasthenia gravis

◆ Disease that causes sporadic but progressive weakness and ab-
normal fatigability of striated (skeletal) muscles
◆ Typically affects muscles innervated by cranial nerves (face,
lips, tongue, neck, throat), but may affect any muscle group
◆ Symptoms exacerbated by exercise and repeated movement
◆ Onset typically between ages 20 and 40
◆ More common among women in this age-group (over age 40,
incidence is similar in men)

**THE PATHO PICTURE**

### UNDERSTANDING MYASTHENIA GRAVIS

During normal neuromuscular transmission, a motor nerve impulse travels to a
motor nerve terminal, stimulating release of a chemical neurotransmitter called
acetylcholine (ACh). When ACh diffuses across the synapse, receptor sites in the
motor end plate react and depolarize the muscle fiber. Depolarization spreads
through the muscle fiber, causing muscle contraction.

In myasthenia gravis, antibodies attach to the ACh receptor sites. They block,
destroy, and weaken these sites, leaving them insensitive to ACh, thereby blocking neuromuscular transmission.

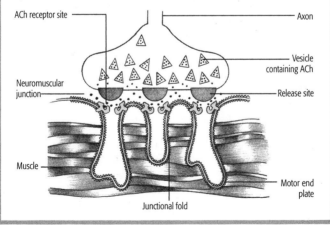

## Causes

◆ Exact cause unknown
◆ May result from autoimmune response, ineffective acetylcholine release, or inadequate muscle fiber response to acetylcholine

## ▲ *Pathophysiologic changes*

| | |
|---|---|
| Impaired neuromuscular transmission to cranial nerves supplying eye muscles ➡ | Weak eye closure, ptosis, diplopia |
| Impaired neuromuscular transmission to skeletal muscles ➡ | Skeletal muscle weakness and fatigue<br>– increase through day; decrease with rest<br>– early stages: easy fatigability of certain muscles (may appear with no other findings)<br>– late stage: may be severe enough to cause paralysis<br>– progressive muscle weakness and accompanying loss of function: depends on muscle group affected; becomes more intense during menses and after emotional stress, prolonged exposure to sunlight or cold, or infections |
| Impaired transmission of cranial nerves innervating facial muscles ➡ | Blank, expressionless facial appearance; nasal vocal tones |
| Cranial nerve involvement ➡ | Frequent nasal regurgitation of fluids; difficulty chewing and swallowing |
| Weakened facial and extraocular muscles ➡ | Drooping eyelids |
| Impaired neuromuscular transmission to diaphragm ➡ | Difficulty breathing, predisposition to pneumonia and other respiratory tract infections |

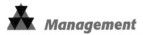

## Management

- Anticholinesterase drugs — *to counteract fatigue and muscle weakness*
- Immunosuppressant therapy (corticosteroids, azathioprine, cyclosporine, and cyclophosphamide, used progressively) — *to decrease immune response toward acetylcholine receptors at neuromuscular junction*
- Immunoglobulin G (during acute relapses) or plasmapheresis (in severe exacerbations) — *to suppress immune system*
- Thymectomy — *to remove thymomas and induce remission in adult-onset myasthenia*
- Tracheotomy, positive-pressure ventilation, and vigorous suctioning — *to improve respiratory function and remove secretions for treatment of acute exacerbations*
- Immediate hospitalization, vigorous respiratory support, discontinuation of anticholinesterase drugs — *for myasthenic crisis, until respiratory function improves*
- Referral to Myasthenia Gravis Foundation — *for information and support*

# Parkinson's disease

◆ Degenerative disease
◆ Produces progressive muscle rigidity, akinesia, and involuntary tremor

**THE PATHO PICTURE**

## NEUROTRANSMITTER ACTION IN PARKINSON'S DISEASE

Parkinson's disease is a degenerative process involving the dopaminergic neurons in the substantia nigra (the area of the basal ganglia that produces and stores the neurotransmitter dopamine). Dopamine deficiency prevents affected brain cells from performing their normal inhibitory function. Other nondopaminergic receptors may be affected, possibly contributing to depression and other nonmotor symptoms.

Dendrite

Axon
Synapse

Dopamine

Receptor
Nerve impulse
Monoamine oxidase B

**Dopamine levels**

Normal level

Lower level

## *Causes*

◆ Unknown
◆ Possibly caused by dopamine deficiency, which prevents affected brain cells from performing normal inhibitory functions in central nervous system
◆ May result from exposure to toxins (manganese dust, carbon monoxide)

### ▲ *Pathophysiologic changes*

| | |
|---|---|
| Loss of inhibitory dopamine activity at synapse ▶ | Cardinal symptoms:<br>– muscle rigidity<br>– akinesia<br>– insidious tremor beginning in fingers (unilateral pill-roll tremor); increases during stress or anxiety and decreases with purposeful movement and sleep |
| Depletion of dopamine ▶ | Muscle rigidity with resistance to passive muscle stretching; may be uniform (lead-pipe rigidity) or jerky (cogwheel rigidity); high-pitched, monotone voice; mask-like facial expression; loss of posture control |
| Impaired regulation of motor function ▶ | Drooling |
| Autonomic dysfunction ▶ | Dysarthria, dysphagia (or both); excessive sweating; decreased motility of gastrointestinal and genitourinary smooth muscle |
| Impaired vascular smooth muscle response ▶ | Orthostatic hypotension |
| Inappropriate androgen production ▶ | Oily skin |

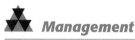 *Management*

- ◆ Levodopa (most effective during early stages; given in increasing doses until symptoms are relieved or side effects appear; usually given in combination with carbidopa) — *to halt peripheral dopamine synthesis*
- ◆ Dopamine agonists (may be used early in disease or in combination with levodopa) — *to enhance response or decrease adverse effects*
- ◆ Alternative drug therapy (anticholinergics, antihistamines, amantadine, or selegiline) when levodopa is ineffective — *to conserve dopamine and enhance therapeutic effect of levodopa*
- ◆ Stereotactic neurosurgery (most effective in younger patients) — *to prevent involuntary movement*
- ◆ Deep brain stimulation (alternative for patients who fail conventional treatment) — *to decrease tremors and allow normal function*
- ◆ Fetal cell transplantation — *to possibly enable brain to process dopamine, halting or reducing disease progression*
- ◆ Active and passive range-of-motion exercises, daily activities, walking, and massage — *to help relax muscles*
- ◆ Complement drug treatment and neurosurgery — *to maintain normal muscle tone and function*
- ◆ Referral to National Parkinson Foundation or United Parkinson Foundation — *for information and support*

# Stroke

- Sudden impairment of cerebral circulation in one or more blood vessels
- Symptoms vary according to affected artery, severity of damage, and extent of collateral circulation
- Stroke in one hemisphere causes features on opposite side of body
- Stroke that damages cranial nerves affects structures on same side of body

**◆ THE PATHO PICTURE**

## UNDERSTANDING STROKE

Strokes are typically classified as ischemic or hemorrhagic, depending on the underlying cause. In either type of stroke, the patient is deprived of oxygen and nutrients.

### Ischemic stroke

This type of stroke results from a blockage or reduction of blood flow to an area of the brain. The blockage may result from atherosclerosis or blood clot formation.

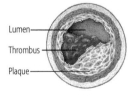

**Common sites of plaque formation**

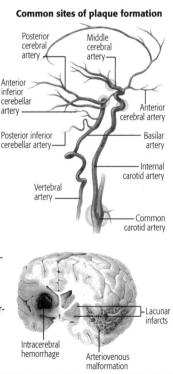

### Hemorrhagic stroke

This type of stroke is caused by bleeding within and around the brain. Bleeding that fills the spaces between the brain and the skull (called subarachnoid hemorrhage) is caused by ruptured aneurysms, arteriovenous malformation, and head trauma. Bleeding within the brain tissue itself (known as intracerebral hemorrhage) is primarily caused by hypertension.

## Causes

- ◆ Thrombosis or emboli (ischemic stroke)
- ◆ Spontaneous bleeding in brain (hemorrhagic stroke)

## Risk factors

- ◆ Hypertension, cardiac disease
- ◆ Family history of stroke
- ◆ History of transient ischemic attacks (TIAs)
- ◆ Diabetes, hyperlipidemia
- ◆ Cigarette smoking, increased alcohol intake
- ◆ Obesity, sedentary lifestyle
- ◆ Use of hormonal contraceptives

## Pathophysiologic changes

| | |
|---|---|
| Thrombosis or hemorrhage of middle cerebral artery ➡ | Aphasia, dysphasia; visual field deficits; hemiparesis of affected side (more severe in face, arm) |
| Thrombosis or hemorrhage of carotid artery ➡ | Weakness, paralysis, numbness; sensory changes; altered level of consciousness; bruits over carotid artery; headaches |
| Thrombosis or hemorrhage of vertebrobasilary artery ➡ | Weakness, paralysis; numbness around lips and mouth; visual field deficits, diplopia, nystagmus; poor coordination, dizziness; dysphagia, slurred speech; amnesia; ataxia |
| Thrombosis or hemorrhage of anterior cerebral artery ➡ | Confusion; weakness, numbness; urinary incontinence; impaired motor and sensory functions; personality changes |
| Thrombosis or hemorrhage of posterior cerebral artery ➡ | Visual field deficits; sensory impairment; dyslexia; cortical blindness; coma |

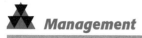

# Management

- ICP monitoring, hyperventilation, osmotic diuretics (mannitol), and corticosteroids (dexamethasone) — *to prevent further cerebral damage*
- Stool softeners — *to prevent straining, which increases ICP*
- Anticonvulsants — *to treat or prevent seizures*
- Surgery (for large cerebellar infarction) — *to remove infarcted tissue and decompress remaining live tissue*
- Aneurysm repair — *to prevent further hemorrhage*
- Percutaneous transluminal angioplasty or stent insertion — *to open occluded vessels*

### FOR ISCHEMIC STROKE

- Thrombolytic therapy (tPA, alteplase [Activase]) within first 3 hours after onset of symptoms — *to dissolve clot, remove occlusion, and restore blood flow, minimizing cerebral damage*
- Anticoagulant therapy (heparin, warfarin) — *to maintain vessel patency and prevent further clot formation*

### FOR TIAS

- Antiplatelet agents — *to reduce risk of platelet aggregation and subsequent clot formation*
- Carotid endarterectomy — *to open partially (greater than 70%) occluded carotid arteries*

### FOR HEMORRHAGIC STROKE

- Analgesics — to relieve headache associated with hemorrhagic stroke

# West Nile encephalitis

- ◆ Vector-borne infectious disease that primarily causes encephalitis (inflammation) of brain
- ◆ Caused by West Nile virus (WNV), a flavivirus (type of mosquito- or tickborne virus that causes yellow fever and malaria) commonly found in humans, birds, and other vertebrates
- ◆ Mortality rate ranges from 3% to 15% (higher among elderly population)

**THE PATHO PICTURE**

## UNDERSTANDING WEST NILE ENCEPHALITIS

West Nile encephalitis is a vector-borne disease. The route of transmission is as follows: Birds serve as the reservoir of the virus. They harbor the virus but can't spread it on their own. Mosquitoes serve as the vectors, spreading it from bird to bird and from bird to people. Humans are believed to be the "dead-end hosts" – the virus lives in people and can make them ill, but feeding mosquitoes do not acquire the virus from biting an infected person. Once the pathogen enters the bloodstream, it travels to the brain and causes encephalitis (inflammation of the brain).

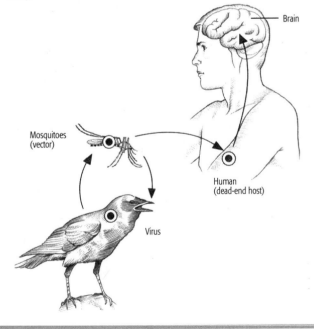

Brain

Mosquitoes
(vector)

Human
(dead-end host)

Virus

## *Causes*

◆ Transmission of WNV through bite by infected mosquito (primarily *Culex* species)
◆ Possible transmission through bite by infected tick

## ▲ *Pathophysiologic changes*

| | |
|---|---|
| Transmission of virus into bloodstream following mosquito bite | Mild infection (most common): <br>– flulike symptoms (fever, headache, body aches) <br>– swollen lymph glands <br>– skin rash |
| Inflammation of brain and spinal cord (occurs as virus travels to neurologic system) | Severe infection (leads to encephalitis): <br>– headache <br>– high fever <br>– neck stiffness <br>– stupor <br>– disorientation <br>– coma <br>– tremors <br>– occasional seizures <br>– paralysis |

## ▲▲ *Management*

◆ Hospitalization — *for severe infection*
◆ I.V. fluids — to maintain adequate hydration
◆ Airway management — to maintain open airway
◆ Ventilator support — to provide adequate oxygenation and ventilation

# 4

# Gastrointestinal disorders

# PATHOPHYSIOLOGIC CONCEPTS

## *Anorexia*

◆ Loss of appetite or lack of desire for food despite normal hunger stimulus (normally stimulated in hypothalamus by falling blood glucose levels)
◆ Can be caused by:
  – slow gastric emptying or gastric stasis
  – high levels of neurotransmitters (such as serotonin)
  – excess cortisol levels (which suppress hypothalamic control of hunger, contributing to satiety)

## *Diarrhea*

◆ Increase in fluidity of feces and frequency of defecation
◆ Characterized by three major mechanisms:
  – osmotic diarrhea (presence of nonabsorbable substance or increased numbers of osmotic particles in intestine increases osmotic pressure and draws excess water into intestine; increases weight and volume of stool)
  – secretory diarrhea (pathogen or tumor irritates muscle and mucosal layers of intestine; consequent increase in motility and secretions [water, electrolytes, mucus] results in diarrhea)
  – motility diarrhea (inflammation, neuropathy, or obstruction causes reflex increase in intestinal motility; may expel irritant or clear obstruction)

## *Jaundice*

◆ Yellow pigmentation of skin and sclera
◆ Results when production of bilirubin exceeds metabolism and excretion and bilirubin accumulates in blood
◆ Occurs when bilirubin levels exceed 2.0 to 2.5 mg/dl

## Nausea

♦ Feeling of urge to vomit
♦ May occur independently of vomiting, or may precede or accompany it
♦ Marked by increased salivation, diminished functional activities of stomach, and altered small intestinal motility
♦ May be stimulated by high brain centers

## Vomiting

♦ Forceful oral expulsion of gastric contents
♦ Occurs when chemoreceptor trigger zone (CTZ) in medulla is stimulated:
  – abdominal muscles and diaphragm contract
  – reverse peristalsis begins, causing intestinal material to flow back into stomach, distending it
  – stomach pushes diaphragm into thoracic cavity, raising intrathoracic pressure
  – pressure forces upper esophageal sphincter open, glottis closes, and soft palate blocks nasopharynx
  – pressure forces material up through sphincter and out through mouth

# DISORDERS

## Cirrhosis

◆ Chronic disease characterized by diffuse destruction and fibrotic regeneration of hepatic cells
◆ Damages liver tissue and normal vasculature
◆ Especially prevalent among malnourished persons over age 50 with chronic alcoholism

**THE PATHO PICTURE**

### UNDERSTANDING CIRRHOSIS

Cirrhosis is a chronic liver disease characterized by widespread destruction of hepatic cells. The destroyed cells are replaced by fibrotic cells in a process called fibrotic regeneration. As necrotic tissue yields to fibrosis, regenerative nodules form, and the liver parenchyma undergo extensive and irreversible fibrotic changes. The disease alters normal liver structure and vasculature, impairs blood and lymphatic flow, and, ultimately, causes hepatic insufficiency.

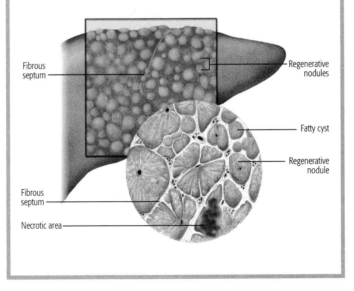

Fibrous septum

Regenerative nodules

Fatty cyst

Regenerative nodule

Fibrous septum

Necrotic area

## *Causes*

◆ Alcoholism
◆ Hepatitis
◆ Biliary obstruction
◆ Hemochromatosis
◆ Budd-Chiari syndrome
◆ Alpha$_1$-antitrypsin deficiency
◆ Wilson's disease

## ▲ *Pathophysiologic changes*

| | |
|---|---|
| Fibrotic changes ➡ | **Hepatomegaly** |
| Gastric stasis ➡ | **Anorexia** |
| Inflammatory response and systemic effects of liver inflammation ➡ | **Nausea and vomiting; dull abdominal ache** |
| Fluid retention ➡ | **Edema and ascities** |
| Impaired liver function ➡ | **Jaundice** |
| Portal hypertension ➡ | **Esophageal varicies** |

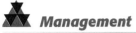

# Management

- Cessation of alcohol ingestion — *to slow progression*
- Vitamins and nutritional supplements — *to improve nutritional status*
- Potassium-sparing diuretics — *to reduce fluid accumulation*
- Rest — *to conserve energy*
- Vasopressin — *to treat esophageal varices*
- Esophagogastric intubation with multilumen tubes — *to control bleeding from esophageal varices or other hemorrhage sites (balloons exert pressure on bleeding site)*
- Paracentesis — *to relieve abdominal pressure and remove ascitic fluid*
- Referral to Alcoholics Anonymous — *to provide support*

# Colorectal cancer

- ◆ Slow-growing cancer that usually starts in inner layer of intestinal tract
- ◆ Commonly begins as polyp
- ◆ Signs and symptoms depend on location of tumor
- ◆ Potentially curable if diagnosed early

**THE PATHO PICTURE**

## HOW COLORECTAL CANCER DEVELOPS

Most lesions of the large bowel are moderately differentiated adenocarcinomas. These tumors tend to grow slowly and remain asymptomatic for long periods. Tumors in the rectum and sigmoid and descending colon grow circumferentially and constrict the intestinal lumen. Tumors in the ascending colon are usually large and palpable.

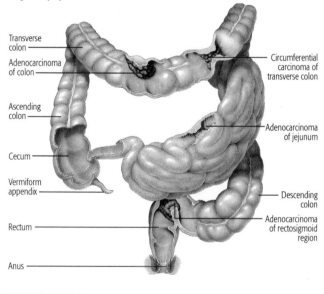

Transverse colon

Adenocarcinoma of colon

Ascending colon

Cecum

Vermiform appendix

Rectum

Anus

Circumferential carcinoma of transverse colon

Adenocarcinoma of jejunum

Descending colon

Adenocarcinoma of rectosigmoid region

## Cause

- ◆ Unknown

## *Risk factors*

◆ Inherited gene mutations
◆ Family or personal history of colorectal cancer
◆ History of intestinal polyps
◆ History of chronic inflammatory bowel disease
◆ Aging
◆ High-fat diet
◆ Obesity and physical inactivity
◆ Diabetes
◆ Smoking
◆ Heavy alcohol intake

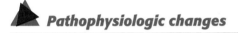

## *Pathophysiologic changes*

### RIGHT SIDE OF COLON
**Early signs**

Gastrointestinal bleeding ▶     Black, tarry stool; anemia

Bowel irritation ▶     Abdominal aching, pressure, or dull cramps

**Late signs**
Anemia ▶     Weakness, fatigue, exertional dyspnea

Intestinal obstruction ▶     Diarrhea, obstipation, anorexia, weight loss, vomiting

### LEFT SIDE OF COLON AND RECTUM
**Early signs**
GI bleeding ▶     Black, tarry stool or rectal bleeding

Intestinal obstruction ▶     Intermittent abdominal fullness or cramping; rectal pressure

**Late signs**
Intestinal obstruction ▶     Obstipation, diarrhea, or "ribbon" or pencil-shaped stool

GI bleeding ▶     Dark or bright red blood in stool and mucus (in or on stool)

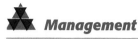

## Management

- ♦ Surgery — *to remove tumor*
  - – Cecum and ascending colon: right hemicolectomy
  - – Proximal and middle transverse colon: right colectomy
  - – Sigmoid colon: Surgery typically limited to sigmoid colon and mesentery
  - – Upper rectum: Anterior or low anterior resection
  - – Lower rectum: Abdominoperineal resection and permanent sigmoid colostomy
- ♦ Chemotherapy — *for patients with metastasis, residual disease, or recurrent inoperable tumor*
- ♦ Radiation therapy (may be used before or after surgery or combined with chemotherapy) — *to induce tumor regression*
- ♦ Referral to enterostomal therapist (if appropriate) — *for stoma management*

# Crohn's disease

◆ Slowly spreading, progressive inflammatory bowel disease
◆ Involves any part of GI tract, usually proximal portion of colon; also may affect terminal ileum
◆ Extends through all layers of intestinal wall
◆ Causes thickening and narrowing of bowel lumen, leading to malabsorption and intestinal obstruction

**THE PATHO PICTURE**

### BOWEL CHANGES IN CROHN'S DISEASE

As Crohn's disease progresses, fibrosis thickens the bowel wall and narrows the lumen. Narrowing (stenosis) can occur in any part of the intestine and cause varying degrees of intestinal obstruction. At first, the mucosa may appear normal, but as the disease progresses it takes on a "cobblestone" appearance, as shown.

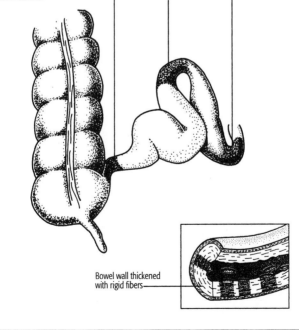

Areas of stenosis

Bowel wall thickened with rigid fibers

## *Causes*

◆ Exact cause unknown
◆ Possibly results from immune reaction to virus or bacterium by causing ongoing intestinal inflammation

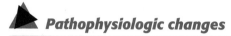 *Pathophysiologic changes*

| | |
|---|---|
| Loss of absorptive surface of functional mucosa ➡ | Protein-calorie malnutrition, dehydration, and nutrient deficiencies; weight loss; diarrhea; steatorrhea |
| Edema of mucosa and bowel spasm ➡ | Obstruction of small or large intestine |
| Bowel spasm ➡ | Steady, colicky pain in right lower quadrant; cramping; tenderness |
| Thickened or matted loops of inflamed bowel ➡ | Palpable mass in right lower quadrant |
| Inflammation ➡ | Bloody stools |

# ▲ *Management*

◆ Corticosteroids — *to reduce inflammation, diarrhea, pain, and bleeding*
◆ Immunosuppressants — *to suppress response to antigens*
◆ Sulfasalazine — *to reduce inflammation*
◆ Infliximab — *to reduce inflammation*
◆ Antidiarrheals — *to combat diarrhea (not used if significant bowel obstruction)*
◆ Opioid analgesics — *to control pain and diarrhea*
◆ Nutritional supplements — *to improve nutritional status*
◆ Dietary modifications (elimination of foods that irritate mucosa or that stimulate excessive intestinal activity) — *to decrease bowel activity while still providing adequate nutrition*
◆ Surgery — *to repair bowel perforation and correct massive hemorrhage, fistulas, or acute intestinal obstruction*

# Diverticular disease

- ◆ Characterized by bulging pouches (diverticula) in GI wall that push mucosal lining through surrounding muscle
- ◆ Classified by two clinical forms:
  - – diverticulosis (diverticula are present but do not cause symptoms)
  - – diverticulitis (diverticula are inflamed; may cause potentially fatal obstruction, infection, or hemorrhage)

**THE PATHO PICTURE**

## HOW DIVERTICULAR DISEASE DEVELOPS

Diverticula probably result from high intraluminal pressure on an area of weakness in the GI wall, where blood vessels enter.

In diverticulitis, retained undigested food and bacteria accumulate in the diverticular sac. This hard mass cuts off the blood supply to the thin walls of the sac, making them more susceptible to attack by colonic bacteria. Inflammation follows and may lead to perforation, abscess, peritonitis, obstruction, or hemorrhage.

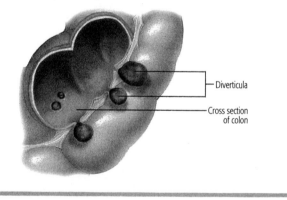

Diverticula

Cross section of colon

## Causes

- ◆ Diminished colonic motility and increased intraluminal pressure
- ◆ Low-fiber diet
- ◆ Defects in colon wall strength

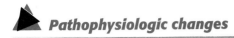 *Pathophysiologic changes*

**MILD DIVERTICULITIS**

Inflammation of diverticula ➡ Moderate left lower abdominal pain

Trapping of bacteria-rich stool in diverticula ➡ Low-grade fever; leukocytosis

**SEVERE DIVERTICULITIS**

Rupture of diverticula and subsequent inflammation and infection ➡ Abdominal rigidity; left lower quadrant pain

Sepsis ➡ High fever, chills, hypotension

Rupture of diverticula near vessel ➡ Microscopic or massive hemorrhage

**CHRONIC DIVERTICULITIS**

Intestinal obstruction ➡ Common signs and symptoms include:
– constipation, ribbon-like stools, intermittent diarrhea
– abdominal distention, rigidity, and pain
– diminishing or absent bowel sounds
– nausea and vomiting

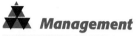 *Management*

♦ Liquid or bland diet, stool softeners, and occasional doses of mineral oil (for symptomatic diverticulosis) — *to maintain bowel function*

♦ High-residue diet (after pain has subsided) — *to help decrease intra-abdominal pressure during defecation*

♦ Exercise — *to increase rate of stool passage*

♦ Antibiotics — *to treat infection of diverticula*

♦ Analgesics — *to control pain and relax smooth muscle*

♦ Antispasmodics — *to control muscle spasms*

♦ Colon resection with removal of involved segment — *to correct cases refractory to medical treatment*

♦ Temporary colostomy — *to drain abscesses and rest colon in diverticulitis accompanied by perforation, peritonitis, obstruction, or fistula*

♦ Thorough patient education about fiber and dietary habits — *to reduce recurrence*

# Gastroesophageal reflux disease

◆ Backflow of gastric or duodenal contents (or both) into esophagus and past lower esophageal sphincter (LES), without associated belching or vomiting
◆ Reflux of gastric contents causes acute epigastric pain, usually after meals

**THE PATHO PICTURE**

## HOW GASTROESOPHAGEAL REFLUX DEVELOPS

Hormonal fluctuations, mechanical stress, and the effects of certain foods and drugs can decrease lower esophageal sphincter (LES) pressure. When LES pressure falls and intra-abdominal or intragastric pressure rises, the normally contracted LES relaxes inappropriately and allows reflux of gastric acid or bile secretions into the lower esophagus. There, the reflux irritates and inflames the esophageal mucosa, causing pyrosis (heartburn).

Persistent inflammation can cause LES pressure to decrease further, possibly triggering a recurrent cycle of reflux and pyrosis.

**Pyrosis**

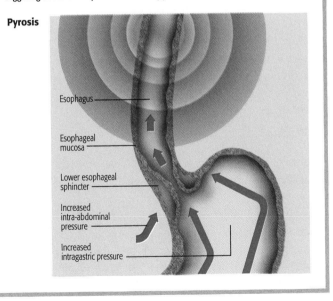

Esophagus

Esophageal mucosa

Lower esophageal sphincter

Increased intra-abdominal pressure

Increased intragastric pressure

## *Causes*

- ◆ Weakened esophageal sphincter
- ◆ Increased abdominal pressure (obesity, pregnancy)
- ◆ Hiatal hernia
- ◆ Medications (morphine, diazepam, calcium channel blockers, meperidine, anticholinergic agents)
- ◆ Food, alcohol, or cigarettes that lower LES pressure
- ◆ Nasogastric intubation for more than 4 days

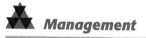 *Pathophysiologic changes*

| Increased abdominal pressure and esophageal irritation ➡ | Burning pain in epigastric area (usually following meals or when lying down) |
|---|---|

## *Management*

- ◆ Dietary modification (frequent, small meals; avoidance of eating before bedtime) — *to reduce abdominal pressure and reduce incidence of reflux*
- ◆ Positioning (sitting up during and after meals; sleeping with head of bed elevated) — *to reduce abdominal pressure and prevent reflux*
- ◆ Increased fluid intake — *to wash gastric contents out of esophagus*
- ◆ Antacids — *to neutralize acidic content and minimize irritation*
- ◆ Histamine-2 receptor antagonists — *to inhibit gastric acid secretion*
- ◆ Proton pump inhibitors — *to reduce gastric acidity*
- ◆ Cholinergic agents — *to increase LES pressure*
- ◆ Smoking cessation or weight loss — *to improve LES pressure*
- ◆ Surgery (if hiatal hernia is cause) — *to repair hiatal hernia*

# Hepatitis, nonviral

- ◆ Inflammation of liver
- ◆ Usually results from exposure to certain chemicals or drugs
- ◆ Complete recovery common; may cause fulminating hepatitis or cirrhosis

**THE PATHO PICTURE**

### EFFECT OF NONVIRAL HEPATITIS ON THE LIVER

After the patient is exposed to a hepatotoxin, hepatic cellular necrosis, scarring, Kupffer cell hyperplasia, and infiltration by mononuclear phagocytes occur with varying severity.

**Nonviral hepatitis**

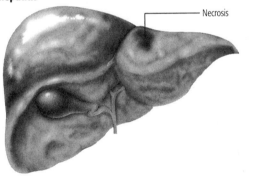

Necrosis

## *Causes*

- ◆ Hepatotoxic chemicals
- ◆ Hepatotoxic drugs

# ▲ *Pathophysiologic changes*

| | |
|---|---|
| Liver inflammation ➡ | Anorexia, nausea, and vomiting; hepatomegaly; possible abdominal pain |
| Decreased bilirubin metabolism ➡ | Jaundice |
| Elevated urobilinogen ➡ | Dark urine |
| Decreased bile in GI tract ➡ | Clay-colored stool |
| Jaundice and hyperbilirubinemia ➡ | Pruritus |

# ▲ *Management*

- ◆ Lavage, catharsis, or hyperventilation (depending on route of exposure) — *to remove causative agent*
- ◆ Acetylcysteine — *as antidote for acetaminophen poisoning*
- ◆ Corticosteroids — *to relieve symptoms of drug-induced nonviral hepatitis*
- ◆ Preventive measures (instructions about proper use of drugs, proper handling of cleaning agents and solvents) — *to prevent recurrence*

# Hepatitis, viral

◆ Common liver infection that causes hepatic cell destruction, necrosis, and autolysis
◆ Major types differentiated by causative virus and transmission
  – Type A (highly contagious; usually results from ingestion of contaminated food or water)
  – Type B (spread through contact with contaminated blood, secretions, and stools)
  – Type C (blood-borne disease associated with shared needles, blood transfusions)
  – Type D (linked to chronic hepatitis B infection; can be severe and lead to fulminant hepatitis)
  – Type E (associated with recent travel to endemic area)

### THE PATHO PICTURE

## EFFECT OF VIRAL HEPATITIS ON THE LIVER

On entering the body, the virus either kills hepatocytes directly or activates inflammatory and immune reactions that injure or destroy the hepatocytes by lysing the infected or neighboring cells. Later, direct antibody attack against the viral antigens causes further destruction of the infected cells. Edema and swelling of the interstitium lead to collapse of capillaries and decreased blood flow, tissue hypoxia, and scarring and fibrosis.

**Viral hepatitis**

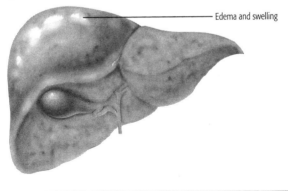

Edema and swelling

## *Cause*

♦ Infection with causative virus

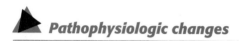

## *Pathophysiologic changes*

### *PRODROMAL STAGE*

| | |
|---|---|
| Systemic effects of inflammation ➡ | Fatigue, malaise, arthralgia, myalgia, fever |
| Anorexia ➡ | Mild weight loss |
| Liver inflammation ➡ | Nausea and vomiting; changes in senses of taste and smell; right upper quadrant tenderness |
| Urobilinogen ➡ | Dark colored urine |
| Decreased bile in GI tract ➡ | Clay-colored stools |

### *CLINICAL STAGE*

Characterized by worsening of all symptoms of prodromal stage as well as the following:

| | |
|---|---|
| Increased bilirubin in blood ➡ | Itching, jaundice |
| Continued liver inflammation ➡ | Abdominal pain or tenderness |

### *RECOVERY STAGE*

Characterized by subsiding of symptoms and return of appetite

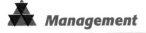

## Management

- Rest — *to minimize energy demands*
- Avoidance of alcohol or other drugs — *to prevent further hepatic damage*
- Dietary modification (small, high-calorie meals) — *to combat anorexia*
- Parenteral nutrition (if patient can't eat due to persistent vomiting) — *to maintain adequate nutritional status*
- Vaccination against hepatitis A and B — *to provide immunity before transmission occurs*
- Enteric precautions (when caring for patients with type A or E hepatitis) — *to prevent spread of infection*
- Supplemental vitamins and feedings — to improve nutritional status

# Irritable bowel syndrome

◆ Benign condition that has no anatomical abnormality or inflammatory component
◆ Marked by chronic symptoms of abdominal pain, alternating constipation and diarrhea, excess flatus, sense of incomplete evacuation, and abdominal distention
◆ Common, stress-related disorder

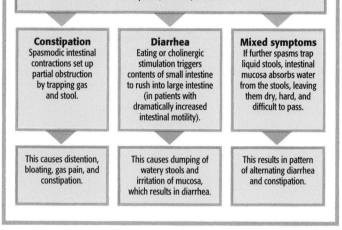

**HOW IT HAPPENS**

Visceral hypersensitivity and altered colonic motility are the mechanisms involved in irritable bowel syndrome (IBS). Some muscles of the small bowel are particularly sensitive to motor abnormalities and distention; others are particularly sensitive to certain foods and drugs. Hypersensitivity to the hormones gastrin and cholecystokinin may also occur. In IBS, the entire colon appears to react to stimuli, causing abnormally strong contractions of the intestinal smooth muscle in response to distention, irritants, or stress.

Autonomic nervous system fails to produce alternating contractions and relaxations that propel stools smoothly toward rectum. This results in constipation, diarrhea, or both.

| **Constipation** | **Diarrhea** | **Mixed symptoms** |
|---|---|---|
| Spasmodic intestinal contractions set up partial obstruction by trapping gas and stool. | Eating or cholinergic stimulation triggers contents of small intestine to rush into large intestine (in patients with dramatically increased intestinal motility). | If further spasms trap liquid stools, intestinal mucosa absorbs water from the stools, leaving them dry, hard, and difficult to pass. |
| This causes distention, bloating, gas pain, and constipation. | This causes dumping of watery stools and irritation of mucosa, which results in diarrhea. | This results in pattern of alternating diarrhea and constipation. |

## *Causes*

- ◆ Pychological stress (most common)
- ◆ Ingestion of irritants (coffee, raw fruit, or vegetables)
- ◆ Lactose intolerance
- ◆ Abuse of laxatives
- ◆ Hormonal changes (menstruation)

## *Pathophysiologic changes*

| | |
|---|---|
| Muscle contraction ➡ | Cramping, lower abdominal pain relieved by defecation or passage of flatus |
| Irritation of nerve fibers by causative stimulus ➡ | Pain that intensifies 1 to 2 hours after a meal |
| Altered colonic movement ➡ | Constipation alternating with diarrhea (one is more dominant); mucus passed through rectum from altered secretion in intestinal lumen; abdominal distention and bloating |

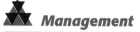 *Management*

◆ Stress-relief measures, counseling, mild anti-anxiety agents — *to improve colon response to stimuli*
◆ Avoidance of food irritants — *to improve colon function*
◆ Application of heat to abdomen — *to relieve spasms and pain*
◆ Antispasmodics — *to treat cramping*
◆ High fiber diet — *to prevent constipation*

### FOR DIARRHEA-DOMINANT IBS

◆ Bulking agents — *to reduce episodes of diarrhea and minimize effect of nonpropulsive colonic contractions*
◆ Loperamide — *to reduce urgency and fecal soiling in patients with persistent diarrhea*
◆ Alosetron (for severe IBS unresponsive to conventional therapy) — *to relieve pain, decrease urgency, and reduce stool frequency*
◆ Bowel training (if cause is chronic laxative abuse) — *to regain muscle control*

### FOR CONSTIPATION-DOMINANT IBS

◆ Cautious use of laxatives — *to prevent dependency on laxative*
◆ Tegaserod (for short-term treatment, usually 4 weeks) — *to facilitate movement of stools through bowel*

# Pancreatitis

- Inflammation of pancreas; occurs in acute and chronic forms
- May be caused by edema, necrosis, or hemorrhage
- Good prognosis when associated with biliary tract disease; poor when associated with alcoholism
- Mortality as high as 60% (with necrosis and hemorrhage)

**THE PATHO PICTURE**

## UNDERSTANDING ACUTE PANCREATITIS

Inflammation of the pancreas may be acute or chronic. Acute pancreatitis, which is life-threatening, may be classified as edematous (interstitial) or necrotizing. In both types, inappropriate activation of enzymes causes tissue damage.

The mechanism that triggers this activation is unknown; however, several conditions are associated with it. The most common include biliary tract obstruction by gallstones and alcohol abuse (alcohol increases stimulation of pancreatic secretions).

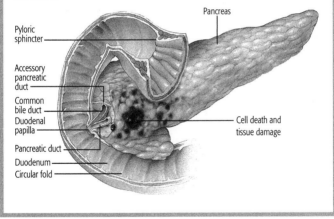

Pancreas

Pyloric sphincter

Accessory pancreatic duct

Common bile duct

Duodenal papilla

Pancreatic duct

Duodenum

Circular fold

Cell death and tissue damage

## *Causes*

◆ Acute pancreatitis:
  – cholelithiasis
  – alcohol abuse
  – abnormal organ structure
  – metabolic or endocrine disorders (hyperlipidemia, hypercalcemia)
  – pancreatic cysts or tumors
  – penetrating peptic ulcers
  – blunt trauma or surgical trauma
  – drugs (glucocorticoids, sulfonamides, thiazides, oral contraceptives)
  – kidney failure or transplantation
◆ Chronic pancreatitis
  – alcohol abuse
  – malnutrition
  – heredity (rare)

## *Pathophysiologic changes*

| | |
|---|---|
| Inflammation ➡ | Midepigastric abdominal pain (can radiate to back); low-grade fever |
| Hypermotility or paralytic ileus secondary to pancreatitis or peritonitis ➡ | Persistent vomiting and abdominal distention (in severe attack) |
| Heart failure ➡ | Crackles at lung bases (in severe attack) |
| Circulating pancreatic enzymes ➡ | Left pleural effusion (in severe attack) |
| Dehydration and possible hypovolemia ➡ | Tachycardia |
| Malabsorption ➡ | Extreme malaise (in chronic pancreatitis) |

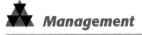 *Management*

- I.V. replacement of fluids, protein, and electrolytes — *to treat imbalances*
- Withholding of food and fluids — *to allow pancreas to rest*
- Antiemetics — *to alleviate nausea and vomiting*
- Meperidine — *to relieve abdominal pain*
- Antacids — *to neutralize gastric secretions*
- Histamine antagonists — *to decrease hydrochloric acid production*
- Antibiotics — *to fight bacterial infections*
- Anticholinergics — *to reduce vagal stimulation, decrease GI motility, and inhibit pancreatic enzyme secretion*
- Insulin — *to correct hyperglycemia*
- Surgical drainage — *to treat pancreatic abscess or pseudocyst or to reestablish drainage of pancreas*
- Laparotomy (if biliary tract obstruction causes acute pancreatitis) — *to remove obstruction*

# 5

# Musculoskeletal disorders

## Pathophysiologic concepts   149

## Disorders   150

# PATHOPHYSIOLOGIC CONCEPTS

## *Altered bone density*

◆ Excess bone resorption that occurs during normal resorption and formation phases of bone remodeling
◆ Decreased estrogen production during early menopause, leading to diminished osteoblastic activity and loss of bone mass
◆ Vitamin D deficiency and inadequate calcium absorption during childhood, which prevents normal bone calcification

## *Altered bone growth*

◆ Insufficient blood supply to growing bones, resulting in avascular necrosis of epiphyseal growth plates (children and adolescents)
◆ Lack of blood to femoral head, leading to septic necrosis and bone softening and resorption
◆ Revascularization, which initiates new bone formation in femoral head or tibial tubercle, causing femoral head malformations

## *Altered bone strength*

◆ Cortical and cancellous bone contribute to skeletal strength
◆ Any loss of inorganic calcium salts constituting chemical structure of bone will weaken bone strength
◆ Cancellous bone is more sensitive to metabolic influences, so conditions that produce rapid bone loss tend to affect cancellous bone more quickly than cortical bone

## *Muscle atrophy*

◆ Decrease in size of muscle tissue or cell
◆ May occur after prolonged inactivity from bed rest or trauma (casting), when local nerve damage makes movement impossible, or when illness robs muscles of needed nutrients
◆ Effects of muscular deconditioning associated with lack of physical activity (reduction of myofibril size) possibly apparent within days

# DISORDERS

## Bone cancer

◆ Osseous bone tumors
 – arise from bony structure itself
 – include osteogenic sarcoma (most common), parosteal osteogenic sarcoma, chondrosarcoma (chondroblastic sarcoma), and malignant giant cell tumor
◆ Nonosseous bone tumors
 – arise from hematopoietic, vascular, and neural tissues
 – include Ewing's sarcoma, fibrosarcoma (fibroblastic sarcoma), and chordoma

**THE PATHO PICTURE**

### UNDERSTANDING OSTEOGENIC SARCOMA

Osteogenic sarcoma, the most common form of bone cancer, arises in osteoid or immature bone, typically involving the long bones of the arms or legs (especially around the knee). Parosteal osteogenic sarcoma arises on the surface of the bone, commonly on the femur near the knee. Chondrosarcoma, which originates in cartilage cells, usually occurs in bones of the pelvis, hip, shoulder, and ribs. Malignant giant cell tumors originate in the epiphyses of the long bones, with most tumors developing in the femur and tibia (some in the humerus and radius).

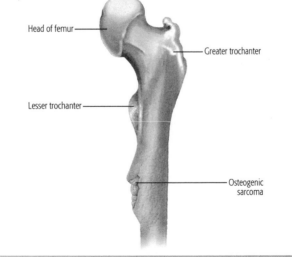

Head of femur

Greater trochanter

Lesser trochanter

Osteogenic sarcoma

## Causes

◆ No immediately apparent cause in most cases
◆ Genetic abnormalities (retinoblastoma, Rothmund-Thomson syndrome)
◆ Carcinogen exposure
◆ Heredity, trauma, excessive radiation therapy

## ▲ Pathophysiologic changes

Inflammation within and around bone ▬▶     Pain

Tumor growth ▬▶     Palpable mass

Weakened bone structure ▬▶     Fractures

## ▲ Management

◆ Tumor excision (along with 1″ margin of bone) and bone grafting or insertion of metal plate — *to remove tumor and maintain function*
◆ External beam radiation — *to eradicate tumor or reduce size*
◆ Brachytherapy (placement of small radioactive pellets directly into tumor) — *to eradicate tumor or reduce size*
◆ Chemotherapy — *to eradicate tumor or reduce size*
◆ Amputation — *when necessary*
◆ Physical therapy — *when assistive devices are necessary*
◆ High-protein, high-calorie diet — *to maintain adequate nutrition*

# Carpal tunnel syndrome

- ◆ Compression of median nerve as it passes through canal (tunnel) formed by carpal bones and transverse carpal ligaments
- ◆ Most common nerve entrapment syndrome

**THE PATHO PICTURE**

### UNDERSTANDING CARPAL TUNNEL SYNDROME

The carpal bones and transverse carpal ligament form the carpal tunnel. Inflammation or fibrosis of the tendon sheaths that pass through the carpal tunnel causes compression and edema of the median nerve. The myelin sheath begins to thin and degenerate. This compression neuropathy causes sensory and motor changes in the median distribution of the hands, initially impairing sensory transmission to the thumb, index finger, second finger, and inner aspect of the third finger.

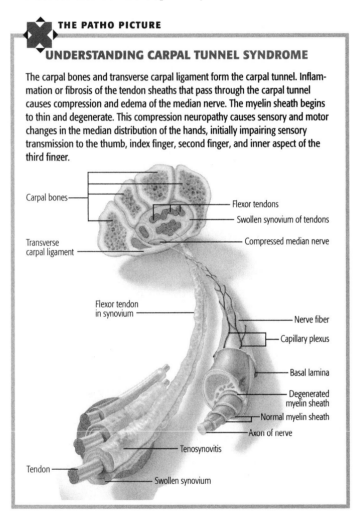

Carpal bones

Flexor tendons
Swollen synovium of tendons

Transverse carpal ligament

Compressed median nerve

Flexor tendon in synovium

Nerve fiber

Capillary plexus

Basal lamina

Degenerated myelin sheath
Normal myelin sheath
Axon of nerve

Tenosynovitis

Tendon

Swollen synovium

## *Causes*

- ◆ Congenital predisposition
- ◆ Trauma or injury to wrist
- ◆ Overactive pituitary gland
- ◆ Hypothyroidism
- ◆ Rheumatoid arthritis
- ◆ Mechanical problems in wrist joint
- ◆ Work-related stress
- ◆ Fluid retention during pregnancy or menopause
- ◆ Development of cyst or tumor within canal
- ◆ Obesity

## *Pathophysiologic changes*

| | |
|---|---|
| Nerve compression ➡ | Weakness, pain, burning, numbness, or tingling of thumb, forefinger, middle finger, and half of fourth finger in one or both hands; inability to clench hand into first |
| Vasodilatation and venous stasis ➡ | Worsening of symptoms at night and in morning |

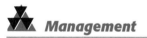

## *Management*

- ◆ Splinting wrist in neutral extension for 1 to 2 weeks — *to rest hand*
- ◆ Nonsteroidal anti-inflammatory drugs — *to relieve symptoms*
- ◆ Injection of carpal tunnel with hydrocortisone and lidocaine — *to provide significant but temporary relief of symptoms*
- ◆ Surgical decompression of nerve by resecting entire transverse carpal tunnel ligament or using endoscopic surgical techniques — *to relieve compression on nerve*
- ◆ Occupational therapy or job retraining if definite link has been established — *to prevent recurrence of symptoms*

# Herniated disk

◆ Protrusion of part of gelatinous center of intervertebral disk (nucleus pulposus) through tear in posterior rim of outer ring (anulus fibrosus)

◆ About 90% occur in lumbar and lumbosacral regions

**THE PATHO PICTURE**

### HOW A HERNIATED DISK DEVELOPS

Physical stress (from severe trauma or strain) or joint degeneration may cause herniation of an intervertebral disk, as shown below.

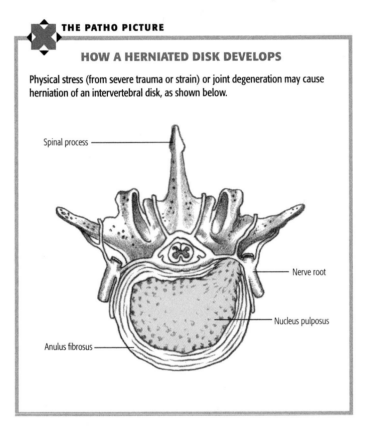

Spinal process

Nerve root

Nucleus pulposus

Anulus fibrosus

## *Causes*

- ◆ Severe trauma or strain
- ◆ Degenerative disk disease

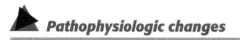 *Pathophysiologic changes*

| | |
|---|---|
| Compression of nerve roots supplying buttocks, legs, and feet ▶ | **Severe low back pain and sciatic pain** |
| Pressure and irritation of sciatic nerve root ▶ | **Muscle spasms** |
| Inactivity ▶ | **Weakness and atrophy of leg muscles (in later stages)** |

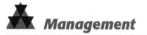 *Management*

- ◆ Heat application — *to diminish muscle spasms and relieve pain*
- ◆ Exercise — *to strengthen associated muscles and prevent further deterioration*
- ◆ Corticosteroids (for initial, short course) and nonsteroidal anti-inflammatory drugs — *to reduce inflammation and edema at injury site*
- ◆ Muscle relaxants — *to minimize muscle spasm from nerve root irritation*
- ◆ Epidural injections at level of protrusion — *to relieve pain*
- ◆ Surgery (laminectomy, spinal fusion) — *to remove extruded disk, overcome segmental instability, and stabilize spine*
- ◆ Supportive care — *to ease discomfort and frustration of chronic lower back pain*

# Osteoarthritis

- ◆ Most common form of arthritis
- ◆ Chronic condition causing deterioration of joint cartilage and formation of reactive new bone at margins and subchondral areas of joints
- ◆ Usually affects weight-bearing joints (knees, feet, hips, lumbar vertebrae)

**THE PATHO PICTURE**

## UNDERSTANDING OSTEOARTHRITIS

Osteoarthritis occurs as synovial joint cartilage deteriorates and reactive, new bone forms at the margins and subchondral areas of the joints. Such degeneration results from damage to chondrocytes (cells responsible for binding cartilage). Cartilage normally softens with age, narrowing the joint space. Mechanical injuries can erode articular cartilage, leaving the underlying bone unprotected. This causes sclerosis (thickening and hardening of the bone beneath the cartilage).

Cartilage flakes irritate the synovial lining, which becomes fibrotic and limits joint movement. Synovial fluid may be forced into defects in the bone, causing cysts. New bone (osteophyte, or bone spur) forms at joint margins as the articular cartilage erodes, causing gross alteration of the bony contours and joint enlargement.

This illustration shows how repeated inflammation results in bony enlargement of the distal interphalangeal and proximal interphalangeal joints of the hand, called Heberden's and Bouchard's nodes.

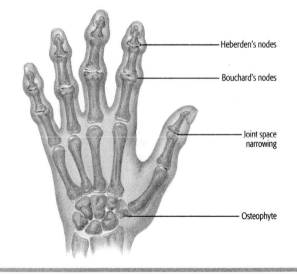

Heberden's nodes

Bouchard's nodes

Joint space narrowing

Osteophyte

## *Causes*

### IDIOPATHIC OSTEOARTHRITIS

◆ Metabolic factors (endocrine disorders, such as hyperparathyroidism) and genetic factors (decreased collagen synthesis)
◆ Chemical factors (drugs that stimulate collagen-digesting enzymes in synovial membrane, such as steroids)
◆ Mechanical factors (repeated stress on joint)

### SECONDARY OSTEOARTHRITIS

◆ Trauma (most common cause)
◆ Congenital deformity
◆ Obesity

## *Pathophysiologic changes*

| | |
|---|---|
| Degradation of cartilage, inflammation, and bone stress (particularly after exercise or weight-bearing activities) ▶ | Deep, aching joint pain (most common symptom, usually relieved by rest); stiffness (in morning and after exercise, usually relieved by rest) |
| Repeated inflammation ▶ | Heberden's nodes (bony enlargements of distal interphalangeal joints) |
| Overcompensation of muscles supporting joints ▶ | Altered gait (from contractures) |
| Pain and stiffness ▶ | Decreased range of motion |
| Bone stress and altered bone growth ▶ | Joint deformity |

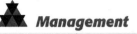 *Management*

◆ Exercise — *to keep joints flexible and improve muscle strength*
◆ Medications (corticosteroids, NSAIDs, Cox-2 inhibitors) — *to control pain*
◆ Glucocorticoid injections — *for inflamed joints unresponsive to nonsteroidal anti-inflammatory agents*
◆ Heat or cold therapy — *for temporary pain relief*
◆ Joint protection — *to prevent strain or stress on painful joints*
◆ Surgery (arthroplasty, arthrodesis, osteoplasty, osteotomy) — *to relieve chronic pain in damaged joints*
◆ Weight control — *to prevent extra stress on weight-bearing joints*

# Osteoporosis

◆ Metabolic bone disorder in which rate of bone resorption accelerates while rate of bone formation slows, causing loss of bone mass

◆ Affected bones lose calcium and phosphate salts, becoming porous, brittle, and abnormally vulnerable to fractures

◆ May be classified as primary disease (often called post-menopausal osteoporosis) or secondary to other causes

**THE PATHO PICTURE**

## HOW OSTEOPOROSIS DEVELOPS

A metabolic bone disorder, osteoporosis develops as the rate of bone resorption accelerates while the rate of bone formation slows, causing a loss of bone mass. Bones weaken as local cells reabsorb bone tissue. Trabecular bone at the core becomes less dense, and cortical bone on the perimeter loses thickness. Bones affected by this disease lose calcium and phosphate salts and become porous, brittle, and abnormally vulnerable to fractures.

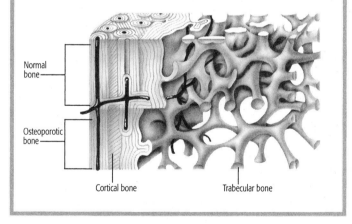

Normal bone

Osteoporotic bone

Cortical bone          Trabecular bone

## Causes

- Unknown (in primary disease), but linked to many risk factors
- Prolonged therapy involving steroids or heparin
- Total immobility or disuse of bone
- Osteogenesis imperfecta
- Medications (aluminum-containing antacids, corticosteroids, anticonvulsants)

## Risk factors

- History of fracture (occurring after age 50)
- Decreased bone mass
- Female (especially postmenopausal)
- Thinness or small body frame
- Advanced age
- Family history of osteoporosis
- Estrogen deficiency (menopause-related)
- Amenorrhea
- Anorexia nervosa
- Low lifetime calcium intake
- Low testosterone level (males)
- Sedentary lifestyle
- Cigarette smoking
- Excessive use of alcohol

## ▲ Pathophysiologic changes

| | |
|---|---|
| Weakened bones ➡ | Loss of height; spinal deformities; spontaneous wedge fractures, pathologic fractures of neck and femur, Colles' fractures of distal radius (common after minor fall), vertebral collapse, and hip fractures |
| Fractures ➡ | Pain |

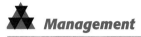 *Management*

♦ Physical therapy (emphasizing gentle exercise and activity) and regular, moderate weight-bearing exercise — *to slow bone loss and possibly reverse demineralization (mechanical stress of exercise stimulates bone formation)*

♦ Supportive devices (back brace) — *to maintain function*

♦ Surgery (if indicated) — *for pathologic fractures*

♦ Hormone replacement therapy (estrogen and progesterone) — *to slow bone loss and prevent fractures*

♦ Analgesics and local heat — *to relieve pain*

♦ Calcium and vitamin D supplements — *to promote normal bone metabolism*

♦ Calcitonin (Calcimar) — *to reduce bone resorption and slow loss of bone mass*

♦ Bisphosphonates (etidronate [Didronel]) — *to increase bone density and restore lost bone*

♦ Fluoride (alendronate [Fosamax]) — *to stimulate bone formation (requires strict dosage, may cause gastric distress)*

♦ Diet rich in vitamin C, calcium, and protein — *to support skeletal metabolism*

# Rhabdomyolysis

◆ Breakdown of muscle tissue
◆ Good prognosis if contributing causes are alleviated or disease is checked before damage becomes irreversible
◆ Unchecked, can cause renal failure

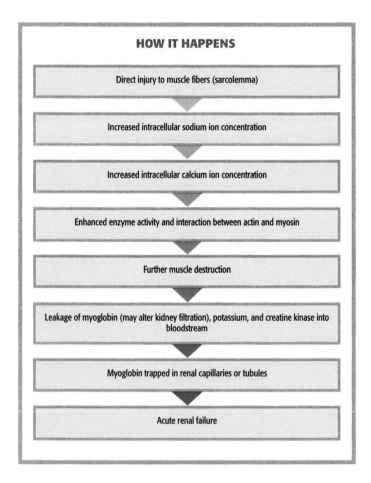

**HOW IT HAPPENS**

Direct injury to muscle fibers (sarcolemma)

Increased intracellular sodium ion concentration

Increased intracellular calcium ion concentration

Enhanced enzyme activity and interaction between actin and myosin

Further muscle destruction

Leakage of myoglobin (may alter kidney filtration), potassium, and creatine kinase into bloodstream

Myoglobin trapped in renal capillaries or tubules

Acute renal failure

## *Causes*

◆ Severe muscle trauma (blunt injury, extensive burns, electrical shock, near drowning)
◆ Excessive muscle activity (status epilepticus, electroconvulsive therapy, severe dystonia)
◆ Familial tendency
◆ Sporadic strenuous exertion (marathon running)
◆ Infection
◆ Medications (antihistamines, salicylates, fibric acid derivatives, HMG-CoA reductase inhibitors, neuroleptics, anesthetics, paralytic agents, corticosteroids, cyclic antidepressants, selective serotonin reuptake inhibitors)

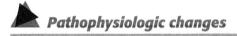 *Pathophysiologic changes*

Muscle trauma and pressure **➡** **Tenderness, swelling, and muscle weakness**

Myoglobin release **➡** **Dark, reddish-brown urine**

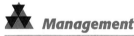 *Management*

◆ Treatment of underlying disorder — *to eliminate cause*
◆ Hydration with I.V. isotonic crystalloid — *to increase intravascular volume and glomerular filtration rate*
◆ Urine alkalinization, osmotic or loop diuretics — *to prevent renal failure*
◆ Analgesics — *for pain*
◆ Immediate fasciotomy and debridement (if compartment syndrome develops and venous pressure is greater than 25 mm Hg) — *to relieve pressure and prevent tissue death*
◆ Exercise modification (prolonged, low-intensity training rather than short bursts of intense exercise) — *to prevent muscle injury and disease*

# 6

# Hematologic disorders

# PATHOPHYSIOLOGIC CONCEPTS

### Red blood cell deficiency (anemia)

♦ Inhibited production of red blood cells (RBCs), marked by increased tissue demand for oxygen (hypoxia); triggers release of erythropoietin (hormone that activates production of RBCs in bone marrow)
♦ Inhibition or destruction of RBCs associated with many factors (drugs, toxins, ionizing radiation, congenital or acquired defects, metabolic abnormalities, deficiency of vitamins or minerals, excessive chronic or acute blood loss, chronic illnesses)

### Red blood cell excess (polycythemia)

♦ Abnormal increase in production of RBCs marked by chronic tissue hypoxia; triggers increased erythropoietin release, excessive RBC production
♦ Decreased plasma volume also causes relative excess of RBCs (often related to dehydration, stress)

### White blood cell deficiency (leukopenia)

♦ Suppressed production of leukocytes, or white blood cells (WBCs), in bone marrow
♦ May be congenital or acquired (drugs, radiation, prolonged stress, systemic disease, viral infection)
♦ Can affect any or all types of WBCs but most commonly neutrophils (predominant type of granular leukocyte, or granulocyte), often resulting in neutropenia
♦ Alters body's defense mechanism, increasing risk of infection; advanced or overwhelming infection may lead to leukopenia

### White blood cell excess (leukocytosis)

♦ Initiated by inflammatory response or infection
♦ Triggers cellular response of phagocytic cells (WBCs that engulf and digest foreign bodies in bloodstream) to site of injury or infection
♦ Mobilization of body's defense mechanism leads to increased WBC production
♦ Pathogenic leukocytosis often associated with cancer and bone marrow disorders

# DISORDERS

## Anemia, folic acid deficiency

◆ Common, slowly progressive, megaloblastic anemia, marked by production of few large, deformed RBCs
◆ Prevalent in infants, adolescents, pregnant and lactating females, alcoholics, elderly, and those with malignant or intestinal diseases

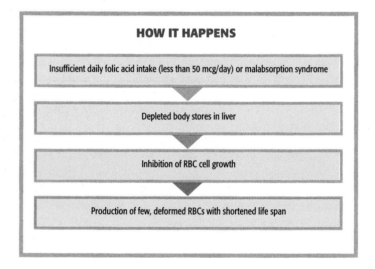

**HOW IT HAPPENS**

Insufficient daily folic acid intake (less than 50 mcg/day) or malabsorption syndrome

Depleted body stores in liver

Inhibition of RBC cell growth

Production of few, deformed RBCs with shortened life span

### Cause

◆ Lack of vitamin folate (folic acid)

### Risk factors

◆ Alcohol abuse
◆ Poor diet
◆ Prolonged drug therapy (anticonvulsants, sulfonamides, and estrogens, including oral contraceptives)
◆ Pregnancy

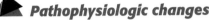 *Pathophysiologic changes*

| | |
|---|---|
| Hypoxemia 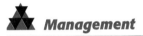 | Progressive fatigue, shortness of breath, palpitations, weakness, pallor |
| Decreased gastrointestinal blood flow ➡ | Nausea, anorexia |
| Decreased blood flow to brain ➡ | Headache, irritability, forgetfulness |

*Management*

◆ Elimination of contributing causes — *to improve metabolism or absorption of folic acid*
◆ Folic acid supplements (orally or parenterally) — *to ensure adequate intake of folic acid*
◆ Well-balanced diet — *to ensure adequate intake of folic acid*

# Anemia, iron deficiency

◆ Oxygen transport disorder characterized by deficiency in hemoglobin synthesis

◆ Most common in premenopausal women, infants (particularly premature or low-birth-weight), children, and adolescents (especially girls)

◆ Favorable prognosis following replacement therapy

**THE PATHO PICTURE**

### UNDERSTANDING
### IRON DEFICIENCY ANEMIA

Iron deficiency anemia occurs when the supply of iron is inadequate for optimal RBC formation, resulting in smaller (microcytic) cells with less color (hypochromic) on staining and, in severe disease, elongated, cigar-shaped cells. Body stores of iron, including plasma iron, become depleted, and the concentration of serum transferrin (which binds with and transports iron) decreases. Insufficient iron stores lead to a depleted RBC mass with subnormal hemoglobin concentration and, in turn, subnormal oxygen-carrying capacity of the blood.

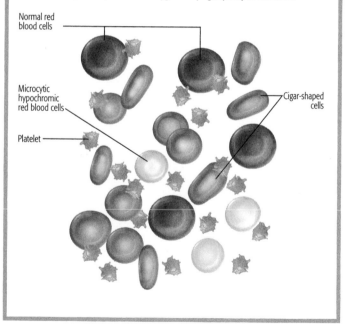

Normal red blood cells

Microcytic hypochromic red blood cells

Platelet

Cigar-shaped cells

## *Causes*

- ◆ Inadequate dietary intake of iron (less than 1 to 2 mg/day), as in prolonged nonsupplemented breast- or bottle-feeding, rapid growth phases
- ◆ Iron malabsorption (chronic diarrhea, partial or total gastrectomy), malabsorption syndromes (celiac disease, pernicious anemia)
- ◆ Blood loss from drug-induced GI bleeding (anticoagulants, aspirin, steroids), heavy menses, traumatic hemorrhage, peptic ulcer, cancer, excessive blood sampling (chronically ill patients), sequestration (dialysis), varices
- ◆ Pregnancy (diverts maternal iron to fetus for erythropoiesis)
- ◆ Intravascular hemolysis-induced hemoglobinuria, paroxysmal nocturnal hemoglobinuria
- ◆ Mechanical trauma to RBCs (prosthetic heart valve, vena cava filter)

## ◢ *Pathophysiologic changes*

| | |
|---|---|
| Decreased oxygen-carrying capacity of blood caused by decreased hemoglobin levels ▶ | Dyspnea on exertion, fatigue, listlessness, pallor, inability to concentrate, irritability, headache, susceptibility to infection |
| Decreased oxygen perfusion ▶ | Increased cardiac output and tachycardia |
| Decreased capillary circulation ▶ | Nails that are coarsely ridged, spoon-shaped (koilonychia), brittle |
| Papillae atrophy ▶ | Sore, red, burning tongue |
| Epithelial changes ▶ | Sore, dry skin at corners of mouth |

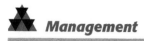 *Management*

♦ Identification of underlying cause — *to permit appropriate treatment of the anemia*
♦ Iron replacement therapy, which may include oral iron preparation (treatment of choice) or combined iron and ascorbic acid (enhances iron absorption) — to ensure adequate intake of iron
♦ Administration of parenteral iron — *for those having problems with oral medication (noncompliance, need for more iron than can be given orally, malabsorption); also given for maximum rate of hemoglobin regeneration*
♦ Careful medication monitoring — *to ensure compliance with prescribed therapy*
♦ Administration of oral supplements at mealtimes— *to decrease gastric irritation*

# Anemia, pernicious

- Most common type of megaloblastic anemia
- Characterized by lack of intrinsic factor (needed to absorb vitamin $B_{12}$) and widespread RBC destruction
- Characteristic manifestations subside with treatment; some neurologic deficits may be permanent

◆ **THE PATHO PICTURE**

### UNDERSTANDING PERNICIOUS ANEMIA

Pernicious anemia is characterized by decreased production of hydrochloric acid in the stomach and a deficiency of intrinsic factor, which is normally secreted by the parietal cells of the gastric mucosa and essential for vitamin $B_{12}$ absorption in the ileum. The resulting vitamin $B_{12}$ deficiency inhibits cell growth, particularly of RBCs, leading to production of few, deformed RBCs with poor oxygen-carrying capacity. RBCs are abnormally large due to excess ribonucleic acid production of the hemoglobin. Pernicious anemia also causes neurologic damage by impairing myelin formation.

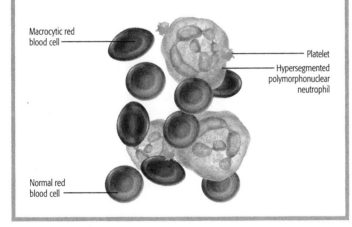

Macrocytic red blood cell

Platelet

Hypersegmented polymorphonuclear neutrophil

Normal red blood cell

## Causes

- Genetic predisposition
- Immunologically related diseases (thyroiditis, myxedema, Graves' disease)
- Partial gastrectomy
- Aging (progressive loss of vitamin $B_{12}$ absorption, usual onset after age 50)

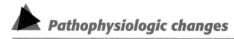
## *Pathophysiologic changes*

### CHARACTERISTIC MANIFESTATIONS

| | |
|---|---|
| Tissue hypoxia ➡ | Weakness |
| Atrophy of papillae ➡ | Sore tongue |
| Interference with nerve impulse transmission (from demyelination) ➡ | Numbness and tingling in extremities |

### OTHER COMMON MANIFESTATIONS

| | |
|---|---|
| Tissue hypoxia ➡ | Pale lips and gums |
| Hemolysis-induced hyperbilirubinemia ➡ | Faintly jaundiced sclera and pale to bright yellow skin |

### GASTRIC ABNORMALITIES

| | |
|---|---|
| Gastric mucosal atrophy and decreased hydrochloric acid production ➡ | Nausea, vomiting, anorexia, weight loss, flatulence, diarrhea, and constipation (from disturbed digestion) |

### NEUROLOGIC ABNORMALITIES

| | |
|---|---|
| Interference of nerve impulse transmission from demyelination (as a result of vitamin B12 deficiency) ➡ | Demyelination initially affects peripheral nerves, but gradually extends to spinal cord, causing various abnormalities: <br> – Lack of coordination; ataxia; impaired fine finger movement <br> – Altered vision (diplopia, blurred vision), taste, and hearing (tinnitus); optic muscle atrophy <br> – Loss of bowel and bladder control; impotence (males) |

### CARDIOVASCULAR ABNORMALITIES

| | |
|---|---|
| Widespread destruction of RBCs caused by increasingly fragile cell membranes ➡ | Low hemoglobin levels |
| Compensatory increased cardiac output ➡ | Palpitations, wide pulse pressure, dyspnea, orthopnea, tachycardia, premature beats, heart failure (eventually) |

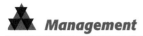

# Management

- Vitamin B$_{12}$ replacement (ongoing for life) — *to ensure adequate intake of B$_{12}$*
- Concomitant iron and folic acid replacement — *to prevent iron deficiency anemia*
- Bed rest — *for extreme fatigue until hemoglobin level rises*
- Blood transfusions — *for dangerously low hemoglobin level*
- Digoxin (Lanoxin), diuretics, low-sodium diet — *to treat heart failure if it occurs*
- Antibiotics — *to combat infection*
- Education materials — *to promote compliance*

# Disseminated intravascular coagulation

◆ Results in small blood vessel occlusion, organ necrosis, depletion of circulating clotting factors and platelets, activation of fibrinolytic system, and consequent severe hemorrhage
◆ Prognosis depends on early detection and treatment, severity of hemorrhage, and treatment of underlying disease

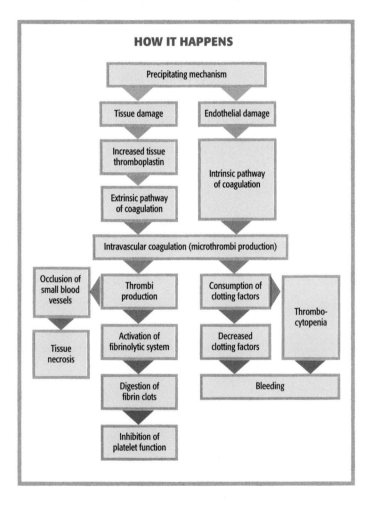

**HOW IT HAPPENS**

Precipitating mechanism

Tissue damage → Increased tissue thromboplastin → Extrinsic pathway of coagulation

Endothelial damage → Intrinsic pathway of coagulation

Intravascular coagulation (microthrombi production)

Occlusion of small blood vessels

Thrombi production

Consumption of clotting factors

Thrombo-cytopenia

Tissue necrosis

Activation of fibrinolytic system

Decreased clotting factors

Digestion of fibrin clots

Bleeding

Inhibition of platelet function

## *Causes*

- ◆ Infection (gram-negative or gram-positive septicemia; viral, fungal, rickettsial, protozoal infections)
- ◆ Obstetric complications (abruptio placentae, amniotic fluid embolism, retained dead fetus, septic abortion, eclampsia)
- ◆ Neoplastic disease (acute leukemia, metastatic carcinoma, aplastic anemia)
- ◆ Disorders that produce necrosis (extensive burns and trauma, brain tissue destruction, transplant rejection, hepatic necrosis)
- ◆ Other possible causes:
  - heatstroke
  - shock
  - poisonous snakebite
  - cirrhosis
  - fat embolism
  - incompatible blood transfusion
  - cardiac arrest
  - surgery requiring cardiopulmonary bypass
  - giant hemangioma
  - severe venous thrombosis
  - purpura fulminans

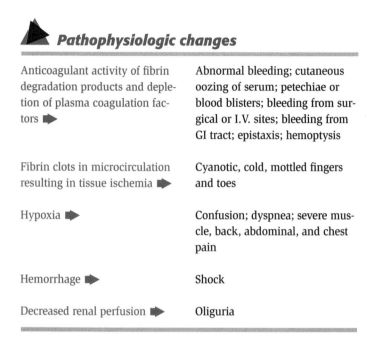

# ▲ *Pathophysiologic changes*

| | |
|---|---|
| Anticoagulant activity of fibrin degradation products and depletion of plasma coagulation factors ➡ | Abnormal bleeding; cutaneous oozing of serum; petechiae or blood blisters; bleeding from surgical or I.V. sites; bleeding from GI tract; epistaxis; hemoptysis |
| Fibrin clots in microcirculation resulting in tissue ischemia ➡ | Cyanotic, cold, mottled fingers and toes |
| Hypoxia ➡ | Confusion; dyspnea; severe muscle, back, abdominal, and chest pain |
| Hemorrhage ➡ | Shock |
| Decreased renal perfusion ➡ | Oliguria |

# ▲▲ *Management*

- ◆ Prompt recognition and treatment of underlying disorder — *to eliminate the cause of DIC*
- ◆ Blood transfusion (fresh frozen plasma, platelet, or packed RBC) — *to support hemostasis in active bleeding*
- ◆ Heparin — *to prevent microclotting (early stages) and treat hemorrhage (as a last resort); controversial in acute coagulation following sepsis*
- ◆ Bed rest — *to prevent injury*
- ◆ Careful monitoring — *to detect new bleeding sites*

# Hodgkin's disease

◆ Neoplastic disorder characterized by painless, progressive enlargement of lymph nodes, spleen, and other lymphoid tissue
from proliferation of various blood cells
◆ Good prognosis with appropriate treatment (5-year survival
rate of about 90%)

**◆ THE PATHO PICTURE**

### UNDERSTANDING HODGKIN'S DISEASE

A neoplastic (tumor-forming) disorder characterized by painless, progressive
enlargement of the lymph nodes, spleen, and other lymphoid tissue, Hodgkin's
disease results from proliferation of lymphocytes, histiocytes, eosinophils, and
Reed-Sternberg giant cells. The hallmark of Hodgkin's disease, Reed-Sternberg
cells (large, binucleated malignant cells found during lymph node biopsy) are
necessary to confirm diagnosis.

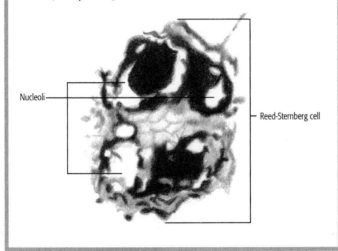

Nucleoli

Reed-Sternberg cell

## *Cause*

◆ Exact cause unknown

## *Risk factors*

- ◆ Genetic factors
- ◆ Age-related factors (peaks in young adulthood, then again in advanced age)
- ◆ Viral factors (linked to Epstein-Barr virus)
- ◆ Environmental factors

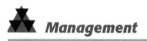

## *Pathophysiologic changes*

| | |
|---|---|
| Proliferation of malignant cells ▶ | Painless swelling of lymph nodes |
| Disease progression ▶ | Fever, night sweats, fatigue; generalized pruritus |
| Lymph node enlargement in the chest ▶ | Cough, chest pain, dyspnea |

## *Management*

- ◆ Radiation therapy — *to kill cancer cells and shrink lymphomas in stage I or II disease*
- ◆ Radiation therapy and chemotherapy (combined therapy) — *to kill cancer cells and shrink lymphomas in stage III disease*
- ◆ Chemotherapy alone (or chemotherapy and radiation therapy to involved sites) — *to kill cancer cells and shrink lymphomas in stage IV disease (sometimes induces complete remission)*
- ◆ Autologous bone marrow transplantation or autologous peripheral blood sternal transfusions and immunotherapy — *to treat Hodgkin's disease that is resistant to standard treatment*
- ◆ Well-balanced diet — *to promote adequate nutritional intake*
- ◆ Frequent rest periods — *to fight fatigue*

# Leukemia

◆ Group of malignant disorders characterized by abnormal proliferation and maturation of lymphocytes and nonlymphocytic cells, leading to suppression of normal cells

◆ Classified as acute or chronic

– Acute lymphocytic leukemia: abnormal growth of lymphocytic precursors (lymphoblasts)

– Acute myelogenous leukemia: rapid accumulation of myeloid precursors (myeloblasts)

– Chronic myelogenous leukemia: abnormal overgrowth of granulocytic precursors (myeloblasts, promyelocytes, metamyelocytes, and myelocytes) in bone marrow, blood, and body tissues

– Chronic lymphocytic leukemia: uncontrollable spread of small, abnormal lymphocytes in lymphoid tissue, blood, and bone marrow

**THE PATHO PICTURE**

### UNDERSTANDING LEUKEMIA

Leukemias cause an abnormal proliferation of WBCs and suppression of other blood components. A rapidly progressing disease, acute leukemia is characterized by the malignant proliferation of WBC precursors (blasts) in bone marrow or lymph tissue and by their accumulation in peripheral blood, bone marrow, and body tissues. In chronic forms of leukemia, disease onset occurs more insidiously, often with no symptoms.

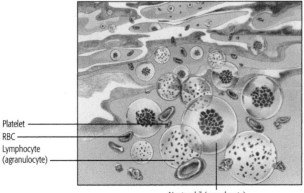

Platelet

RBC

Lymphocyte (agranulocyte)

Neutrophil (granulocyte)

## Cause

◆ Exact cause unknown

## Risk factors

◆ Viral or genetic factors
◆ Exposure to ionizing radiation and chemicals

## ▲ Pathophysiologic changes

**ACUTE LEUKEMIA**

| | |
|---|---|
| Bone marrow invasion and cellular proliferation ➡ | Sudden onset of high fever |
| Anemia ➡ | Fatigue, malaise, dyspnea |
| Thrombocytopenia ➡ | Petechiae, bruising, mucous membrane bleeding, epistaxis |
| Neutropenia ➡ | Fever, possible infection |
| Leukemic infiltration of bone ➡ | Bone and joint pain (acute lymphocytic leukemia) |
| Central nervous system involvement from leukemic infiltration or cerebral bleeding ➡ | Headache, nausea, vomiting, cranial nerve palsy and meningeal irritation (acute lymphocytic leukemia) |

**CHRONIC LEUKEMIA**

| | |
|---|---|
| Anemia ➡ | Slow onset of fatigue, malaise, pallor, and dyspnea |
| Thrombocytopenia ➡ | Petechiae, bruising, mucous membrane bleeding, epistaxis (chronic myelogenous leukemia) |
| Lymphadenopathy, splenomegaly, hepatomegaly ➡ | Abdominal discomfort |
| Neutropenia ➡ | Fever, possible infection |
| Lymphocytic infiltrates ➡ | Skin eruptions |

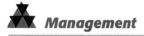

# Management

♦ Systemic chemotherapy (varies according to type of leukemia) — *to eradicate leukemic cells and induce remission*
♦ Bone marrow or stem cell transplants (in some cases) — *to eradicate leukemic cells and induce remission*
♦ Antibiotics, antifungals, antiviral therapy — *to prevent or control infection*
♦ Platelet and red blood cell transfusions — *to treat anemia and prevent bleeding*
♦ Local radiation — *to reduce organ size (when chronic lymphocytic leukemia causes obstruction or organ impairment)*
♦ Psychological support — *to promote communication and trust*
♦ Palliative and supportive care — *for those refractory to chemotherapy or in terminal phase of disease*

# Non-Hodgkin's lymphoma

◆ Malignant lymphoma originating in lymph glands and other lymphoid tissue

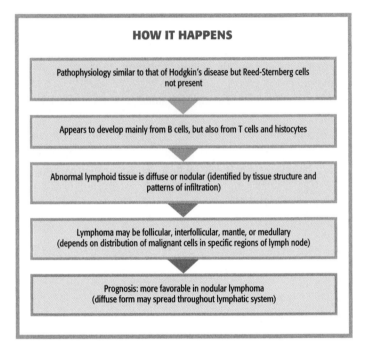

**HOW IT HAPPENS**

Pathophysiology similar to that of Hodgkin's disease but Reed-Sternberg cells not present

Appears to develop mainly from B cells, but also from T cells and histocytes

Abnormal lymphoid tissue is diffuse or nodular (identified by tissue structure and patterns of infiltration)

Lymphoma may be follicular, interfollicular, mantle, or medullary (depends on distribution of malignant cells in specific regions of lymph node)

Prognosis: more favorable in nodular lymphoma (diffuse form may spread throughout lymphatic system)

## Cause

◆ Exact cause unknown

## Risk factors

◆ Genetic factors
◆ Viral factors (linked to Epstein-Barr virus)
◆ Exposure to ionizing radiation and chemicals (herbicides, pesticides, benzene)

# ▲ *Pathophysiologic changes*

| | |
|---|---|
| Cellular proliferation ➡ | Swollen lymph glands; enlarged tonsils and adenoids; painless, rubbery nodes in cervical supraclavicular areas |
| Lymphocytic infiltration of oropharynx and thorax ➡ | Dyspnea and coughing |
| Mechanical obstruction of abdominal tissues ➡ | Abdominal pain and constipation |
| Disseminated disease and extensive tumor growth ➡ | Fatigue, malaise, fever, weight loss, night sweats |

# ▲ *Management*

- ◆ Radiation therapy (mainly in early, localized disease) — *to kill cancer cells and shrink lymphomas*
- ◆ Chemotherapy (most effective with multiple combinations of antineoplastics) — *to kill cancer cells*
- ◆ Bone marrow and stem cell transplants (in some cases, especially following relapse after initial chemotherapy) — *to treat non-Hodgkin's disease that is resistant to standard treatment*
- ◆ Psychological support — *to promote communication and trust*

# Thalassemia

- ◆ Hereditary group of hemolytic anemias
- ◆ Results from defect in protein synthesis of hemoglobin
- ◆ RBC synthesis also is impaired
- ◆ Most common in people of Mediterranean ancestry
- ◆ ß-thalassemia (most common type) occurs in two clinical forms: major and minor

**THE PATHO PICTURE**

### UNDERSTANDING THALASSEMIA

A hereditary group of hemolytic anemias, thalassemia is characterized by defective synthesis in the polypeptide chains of the protein component of hemoglobin. Consequently, RBC synthesis also is impaired.

In thalassemia major, survival to adulthood seldom occurs. In thalassemia minor, a normal lifespan is expected. Severity depends on whether the patient is homozygous or heterozygous for the thalassemic trait.

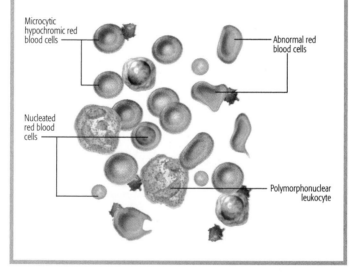

Microcytic hypochromic red blood cells

Abnormal red blood cells

Nucleated red blood cells

Polymorphonuclear leukocyte

## Causes

- ◆ Homozygous inheritance of partially dominant autosomal gene (thalassemia major or intermedia)
- ◆ Heterozygous inheritance of the same gene (thalassemia minor)

# 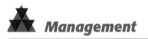 *Pathophysiologic changes*

### THALASSEMIA MAJOR

Mutation in both beta globin
chains of hemoglobin ➡

Underproduction of hemoglobin,
severe anemia, pallor, bone abnormalities, fatigue, failure to
thrive

Infection ➡

Fever

Erythroid hyperplasia and cortical bone thinning ➡

Deformed skull bones

### THALASSEMIA MINOR

Mutation in one beta globin
chain of hemoglobin ➡

Mild anemia (carrier of genetic
trait)

# *Management*

### THALASSEMIA MAJOR

◆ Transfusions (packed RBCs) — *to increase hemoglobin levels
(used judiciously to minimize iron overload)*
◆ Prompt treatment with appropriate antibiotics — *for infections*
◆ Chelation therapy — *to remove excess iron from frequent blood
transfusions*
◆ Bone marrow transplantation — *may be curative in some patients*

### THALASSEMIA MINOR

◆ Patient teaching — *to inform patients that their condition is
hereditary and may be mistaken for iron deficiency anemia*
◆ Genetic counseling (for adults desiring children) — *to provide
pregnancy planning*

# Thrombocytopenia

- ◆ Most common cause of hemorrhagic disorders
- ◆ Deficiency of circulating platelets that may be congenital or acquired (more common)
- ◆ Poses serious threat to hemostasis (platelets are essential for coagulation)

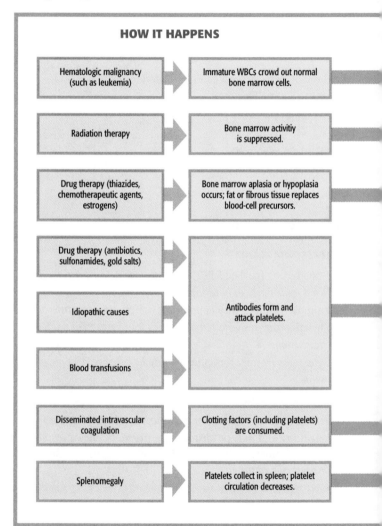

**HOW IT HAPPENS**

| | |
|---|---|
| Hematologic malignancy (such as leukemia) | Immature WBCs crowd out normal bone marrow cells. |
| Radiation therapy | Bone marrow activitiy is suppressed. |
| Drug therapy (thiazides, chemotherapeutic agents, estrogens) | Bone marrow aplasia or hypoplasia occurs; fat or fibrous tissue replaces blood-cell precursors. |
| Drug therapy (antibiotics, sulfonamides, gold salts) | Antibodies form and attack platelets. |
| Idiopathic causes | |
| Blood transfusions | |
| Disseminated intravascular coagulation | Clotting factors (including platelets) are consumed. |
| Splenomegaly | Platelets collect in spleen; platelet circulation decreases. |

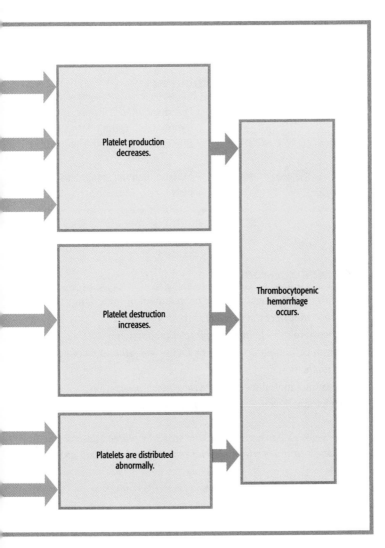

## Causes

♦ Decreased or defective platelet production in bone marrow (leukemia, aplastic anemia, drug toxicity)
♦ Increased platelet destruction outside marrow resulting from underlying disorder (cirrhosis, disseminated intravascular coagulation, or severe infection)
♦ Sequestration (increased amount of blood in limited vascular area, such as spleen)
♦ Blood loss

## Pathophysiologic changes

| | |
|---|---|
| Inadequate hemostasis ➡ | Petechiae; blood blisters; mucous membrane bleeding; large, blood-filled blisters in mouth (adults) |
| Decreased oxygenation ➡ | Malaise, fatigue, general weakness |

## Management

♦ Withdrawal of offending drug or treatment of underlying cause — *to correct the cause of thrombocytopenia*
♦ Corticosteroids — *to increase platelet production*
♦ Lithium carbonate (Eskalith) or folate — *to stimulate bone marrow production*
♦ I.V. gamma globulin — *to increase platelet production*
♦ Platelet transfusion — *to treat complications of severe hemorrhage*
♦ Splenectomy — *to correct disease caused by platelet destruction (spleen is primary site of platelet removal and antibody production)*

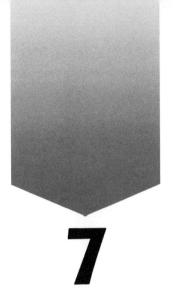

# 7

# Immunologic disorders

# PATHOPHYSIOLOGIC CONCEPTS

## *Autoimmune reactions*

♦ Body's normal defenses become self-destructive, recognizing self-antigens as foreign
♦ Cause unclear; may result from combination of factors (genetic, hormonal, and environmental influences)
♦ Many reactions characterized by B-cell hyperactivity and hyper-gammaglobulinemia (B-cell hyperactivity may be related to T-cell abnormalities)

## *Hypersensitivity*

♦ Exaggerated or inappropriate response occurring on second ex-posure to antigen, leading to inflammation and destruction of healthy tissue
♦ Reactions may be immediate (within minutes to hours of re-exposure) or delayed (several hours after reexposure)
♦ Delayed reaction typically is most severe days after reexposure
♦ Classified by type: type I (mediated by IgE), type II (tissue-specific), type III (immune complex–mediated), type IV (cell-mediated)

### TYPE I HYPERSENSITIVITY

♦ Allergen activates T cells, inducing B-cell production of IgE, which binds to Fc receptors on surface of mast cells
♦ Repeated exposure to relatively large doses of allergen is usual-ly necessary
♦ Sensitization to allergen occurs when enough IgE has been pro-duced
♦ At next exposure, antigen binds with surface IgE, cross-links to Fc receptors, and causes mast cells to degranulate and release various mediators resulting in hypotension, wheezing, swelling, urticaria, and rhinorrhea

### TYPE II HYPERSENSITIVITY

◆ Antibodies directed against cell-surface antigens destroy target cell
◆ Tissue damage occurs through several mechanisms:
  – antigen-antibody binding activates complement, which ultimately disrupts cellular membranes (complement-mediated lysis)
  – phagocytic cells with receptors for immunoglobulin (Fc region) and complement fragments envelop and destroy opsonized targets (red blood cells, leukocytes, platelets)
  – cytotoxic T cells and natural killer cells (not antigen-specific in themselves) damage tissue by releasing toxic substances that destroy cells
  – antibody binding causes malfunction, not destruction, of target cell

### TYPE III HYPERSENSITIVITY

◆ Circulating antigen-antibody complexes (immune complexes) accumulate and deposit in tissues (kidneys, joints, skin, blood vessels)
◆ Complement cascade is activated, causing local inflammation
◆ Platelet release of vasoactive amines is triggered, causing increased vascular permeability and accumulation of immune complexes in vessel walls
◆ Complement fragments attract neutrophils
◆ Neutrophils attempt to unsuccessfully ingest immune complexes and release lysosomal enzymes, which exacerbate tissue damage

### TYPE IV HYPERSENSITIVITY

◆ Antigen-presenting cells bring antigen to T cells
◆ Sensitized T cells release lymphokines, which stimulate macrophages
◆ Lysozymes are released, and surrounding tissue is damaged

# DISORDERS

## Acquired immunodeficiency syndrome (AIDS)

◆ Acquired through blood or body-fluid transmission of human immunodeficiency virus (HIV)
◆ Characterized by gradual destruction of cell-mediated (T cell) immunity and autoimmunity, causing susceptibility to opportunistic infections, cancer, and other abnormalities
◆ Diagnosis based on HIV status and presence of fewer than 200 CD4$^+$ T cells per cubic millimeter of blood

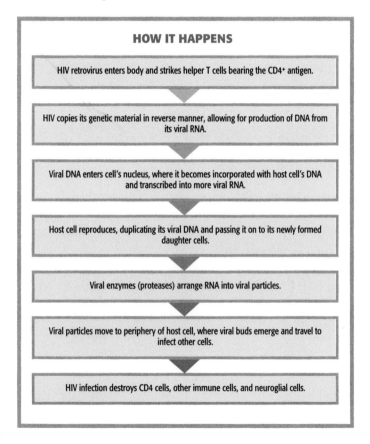

**HOW IT HAPPENS**

HIV retrovirus enters body and strikes helper T cells bearing the CD4$^+$ antigen.

HIV copies its genetic material in reverse manner, allowing for production of DNA from its viral RNA.

Viral DNA enters cell's nucleus, where it becomes incorporated with host cell's DNA and transcribed into more viral RNA.

Host cell reproduces, duplicating its viral DNA and passing it on to its newly formed daughter cells.

Viral enzymes (proteases) arrange RNA into viral particles.

Viral particles move to periphery of host cell, where viral buds emerge and travel to infect other cells.

HIV infection destroys CD4 cells, other immune cells, and neuroglial cells.

## *Cause*
◆ Contact with HIV-infected blood or body fluids (HIV-1 or HIV–2)

## *Risk factors*
◆ Sharing drug needles or syringes
◆ Sexual contact with HIV-infected person without use of condom
◆ Sexual contact with person with unknown HIV status

## ◢ *Pathophysiologic changes*

| | |
|---|---|
| Altered function of CD4$^+$ cells, immunodeficiency, and infection of other CD4$^+$ antigen–bearing cells ▶ | Persistent generalized lymphadenopathy; weight loss, fatigue, night sweats, fever |
| HIV encephalopathy and infection of neuroglial cells ▶ | Neurologic symptoms (forgetfulness, imbalance, weakness, impaired language) |
| Immunodeficiency ▶ | Opportunistic infection (such as cytomegalovirus) or cancer (such as Kaposi's sarcoma) |

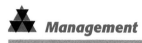

## Management

- Primary therapy: combination of three different types of anti-retroviral agents — *to inhibit HIV viral replication with fewest adverse reactions*
- Current recommendations: use of two nucleosides (interfere with copying of viral RNA into DNA by reverse transcriptase) plus one protease inhibitor (block replication of virus particle and reduce number of new virus particles produced), or two nucleosides and one nonnucleoside (interfere with action of reverse transcriptase) — *to inhibit production of resistant, mutant strains*
- Immunomodulatory agents — *to boost immune system weakened by AIDS and retroviral therapy*
- Human granulocyte colony-stimulating growth factor — *to stimulate neutrophil production (retroviral therapy causes anemia, so patients may receive epoetin alfa)*
- Anti-infective and antineoplastic agents — *to combat opportunistic infections and associated cancers (some prophylactically to help resist opportunistic infections)*
- Supportive therapy (nutritional support, fluid and electrolyte replacement therapy, pain relief, psychological support) — *to provide comfort*
- Diligent practice of standard precautions — *to prevent inadvertent transmission of AIDS and other infectious diseases transmitted by similar routes*
- Information about AIDS societies and support programs — *to educate patient and significant others*

# Anaphylaxis

◆ Acute, potentially life-threatening type I (immediate) hypersensitivity reaction marked by sudden onset of rapidly progressive urticaria (vascular swelling in skin accompanied by itching) and respiratory distress

◆ Occurs within minutes but can occur up to 1 hour after reexposure to antigen

⬧ **THE PATHO PICTURE**

## UNDERSTANDING ANAPHYLAXIS

### 1. Response to antigen
Immunoglobulins (Ig) M and G recognize and bind to antigen.

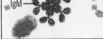

Complement cascade

### 2. Release of chemical mediators
Activated IgE on basophils promotes release of mediators: histamine, serotonin, and leukotrienes.

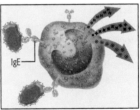

Histamine **H**   Serotonin ◆   Leukotrienes ✳

### 3. Intensified response
Mast cells release more histamine and eosinophil chemotactic factor of anaphylaxis (ECF-A), which create venule-weakening lesions.

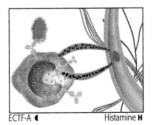

ECTF-A ◀                    Histamine **H**

*(continued)*

**THE PATHO PICTURE**

## UNDERSTANDING ANAPHYLAXIS *(continued)*

### 4. Respiratory distress

In the lungs, histamine causes endothelial cell destruction and fluid leakage into alveoli.

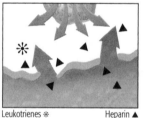

Leukotrienes ✳          Histamine **H**

### 5. Deterioration

Meanwhile, mediators increase vascular permeability, causing fluid leak from the vessels.

Bradykinin ●          Prostaglandins +
Histamine **H**          Serotonin ◆

### 6. Failure of compensatory mechanisms

Endothelial cell damage causes basophils and mast cells to release heparin and mediator-neutralizing substances. However, anaphylaxis is now irreversible.

Leukotrienes ✳          Heparin ▲

## Causes

◆ Ingestion of (or systemic exposure to) sensitizing drugs or other substances:
  – serums (horse serum), vaccines, allergen extracts
  – penicillin or other antibiotics, sulfonamides, local anesthetics
  – diagnostic chemicals (sulfobromophthalein sodium, sodium dehydrocholate, radiographic contrast media)
  – food proteins (legumes, nuts, berries, seafood, egg albumin)
  – sulfite-containing food additives
  – insect venom

# ▲ *Pathophysiologic changes*

| | |
|---|---|
| Activation of IgE and subsequent release of chemical mediators ▶ | Feeling of impending doom or fright |
| Histamine release ▶ | Sweating; sneezing, shortness of breath, nasal pruritus, urticaria, and angioedema (swelling of nerves and blood vessels); nasal mucosal edema; profuse watery rhinorrhea; itching; nasal congestion |
| Increased vascular permeability, subsequent decrease in peripheral resistance and leakage of plasma fluids ▶ | Hypotension, shock, and cardiac arrhythmias (sometimes) |
| Increased capillary permeability and mast cell degranulation ▶ | Edema of upper respiratory tract, resulting in hypopharyngeal and laryngeal obstruction |
| Bronchiole smooth muscle contraction and increased mucus production ▶ | Hoarseness, stridor, wheezing, and accessory muscle use |
| Smooth muscle contraction of intestines and bladder ▶ | Severe stomach cramps, nausea, diarrhea; urinary urgency and incontinence |

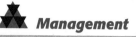 *Management*

- Immediate administration of epinephrine 1:1,000 aqueous solution (I.M. or subcutaneously if patient hasn't lost consciousness and is normotensive; I.V. if reaction is severe), repeating dosage every 5 to 20 minutes as needed — *to reverse bronchoconstriction and cause vasoconstriction*
- Tracheostomy or endotracheal intubation and mechanical ventilation — *to maintain patent airway*
- Oxygen therapy — *to increase tissue perfusion*
- Longer-acting epinephrine, corticosteroids, diphenhydramine (Benadryl) — *to reduce allergic response (long-term management)*
- Albuterol mini-nebulizer treatment — *to reverse bronchospasm*
- Histamine-2 blocker — *to reduce histamine release*
- Aminophylline — *to reverse bronchospasm*
- Volume expanders — *to maintain and restore circulating plasma volume*
- I.V. vasopressors (norepinephrine, dopamine) — *to stabilize blood pressure*
- Cardiopulmonary resuscitation — *to treat cardiac arrest*

# Rheumatoid arthritis

◆ Chronic, systemic inflammatory disease that primarily attacks peripheral joints and surrounding muscles, tendons, ligaments, and blood vessels
◆ Characterized by partial remissions and unpredictable exacerbations

**THE PATHO PICTURE**

## UNDERSTANDING RHEUMATOID ARTHRITIS

A potentially crippling disease, rheumatoid arthritis primarily attacks peripheral joints and surrounding tissues through chronic inflammation. If not arrested, the inflammatory process occurs in four stages:

◆ Synovitis develops from congestion and edema of the synovial membrane and joint capsule. Infiltration by lymphocytes, macrophages, and neutrophils continues the local inflammatory response. These cells, as well as fibroblast-like synovial cells, produce enzymes that help degrade bone and cartilage.
◆ Pannus (thickened layers of granulation tissue) covers and invades cartilage, eventually destroying the joint capsule and bone.
◆ Fibrous ankylosis (fibrous invasion of the pannus and scar formation) occludes the joint space. Bone atrophy and misalignment cause visible deformities and disrupt the articulation of opposing bones, resulting in muscle atrophy and imbalance and, possibly, partial dislocations (subluxations).
◆ Fibrous tissue calcifies, resulting in bony ankylosis and total immobility.

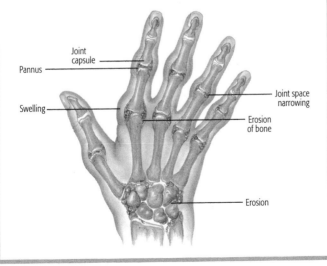

## *Cause*

♦ Unknown

## ▲ *Pathophysiologic changes*

| | |
|---|---|
| Initial inflammatory reactions before inflammation of synovium ▶ | Fatigue, malaise, anorexia and weight loss, persistent low-grade fever, lymphadenopathy, vague articular symptoms |
| Prostaglandin release; inflammation and destruction of synovium ▶ | Specific localized, bilateral, and symmetric articular symptoms (in fingers at proximal interphalangeal, metacarpophalangeal, and metatarsophalangeal joints; may extend to wrists, knees, elbows, and ankles); stiffening of affected joints after inactivity (especially on arising in morning); spindle-shaped fingers; joint pain and tenderness; feeling of warmth at joint; rheumatoid nodules |
| Swelling and loss of joint space ▶ | Flexion deformities or hyperextension of metacarpophalangeal joints; subluxation of the wrist; stretching of tendons, pulling fingers to ulnar side (ulnar drift); characteristic swan-neck or boutonnière deformity |
| Infiltration of nerve fibers ▶ | Peripheral neuropathy (numbness or tingling in feet, weakness and loss of sensation in fingers) |

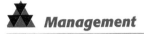 *Management*

♦ Salicylates, particularly aspirin (mainstay of therapy) — *to decrease inflammation and relieve joint pain*
♦ Nonsteroidal anti-inflammatory agents, such as fenoprofen (Nalfon), ibuprofen (Motrin), and indomethacin (Indocin) — *to relieve inflammation and pain*
♦ Antimalarials such as hydroxychloroquine sulfate (Plaquenil), sulfasalazine (Azulfidine), gold salts, and penicillamine (Cuprimine) — *to reduce acute and chronic inflammation*
♦ Corticosteroids (prednisone) — *for anti-inflammatory effects (low doses), for immunosuppressive effect on T cells (higher doses)*
♦ Azathioprine (Imuran), cyclosporine (Neoral), methotrexate (Folex) in early disease — *for immunosuppression (suppresses T and B lymphocyte proliferation, which destroys synovium)*
♦ Synovectomy (removal of destructive, proliferating synovium, usually in wrists, knees, and fingers) — *to possibly halt or delay disease course*
♦ Osteotomy (cutting of bone or excision of bone wedge) — *to re-align joint surfaces and redistribute stress*
♦ Tendon transfers — *to prevent deformities or relieve contractures*
♦ Joint reconstruction or total joint arthroplasty (including metatarsal head and distal ulnar resectional arthroplasty, insertion of a Silastic prosthesis between metacarpophalangeal and proximal interphalangeal joints) — *to treat and correct deformities in severe disease*
♦ Arthrodesis (joint fusion) — *for stability and pain relief (sacrifices joint mobility)*

# Scleroderma

◆ Diffuse autoimmune connective tissue disease
◆ Characterized by inflammatory, degenerative, and fibrotic changes in skin, blood vessels, synovial membranes, skeletal muscles, and internal organs
◆ May be localized (skin and musculoskeletal system) or generalized (skin, musculoskeletal system, and internal organs)
◆ Slowly progressing, uncommon disease that affects mostly women (three to four times more than men)

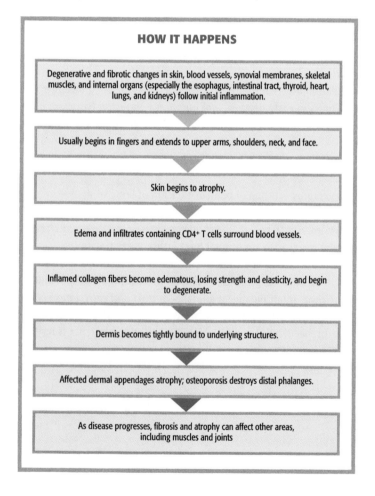

**HOW IT HAPPENS**

Degenerative and fibrotic changes in skin, blood vessels, synovial membranes, skeletal muscles, and internal organs (especially the esophagus, intestinal tract, thyroid, heart, lungs, and kidneys) follow initial inflammation.

Usually begins in fingers and extends to upper arms, shoulders, neck, and face.

Skin begins to atrophy.

Edema and infiltrates containing CD4+ T cells surround blood vessels.

Inflamed collagen fibers become edematous, losing strength and elasticity, and begin to degenerate.

Dermis becomes tightly bound to underlying structures.

Affected dermal appendages atrophy; osteoporosis destroys distal phalanges.

As disease progresses, fibrosis and atrophy can affect other areas, including muscles and joints

## *Cause*

◆ Unknown

## *Pathophysiologic changes*

| | |
|---|---|
| Excess collagen deposited in skin ▶ | Skin changes:<br>– hardening and thickening of skin<br>– ulcers or sores on fingers<br>– loss of hair over affected area<br>– change in skin color<br>– swelling, puffiness in fingers and toes<br>– shiny skin<br>– disappearance of skin creases |
| Damage to small blood vessels ▶ | Raynaud's phenomenon |
| Calcium deposits ▶ | Calcinosis |
| Excess collagen in joints and muscles ▶ | Arthritis and muscle weakness |
| Loss of lower esophageal sphincter function ▶ | Frequent reflux, heartburn, dysphagia, and bloating after meals |
| Scarring of organs or thickening of blood vessels ▶ | Heart or kidney failure, interstitial lung disease, pulmonary hypertension |

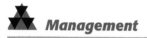

## Management

- Nonsteroidal anti-inflammatory agents — *for inflammation and pain*
- Immunosuppressants — *to decrease skin thickening and improve other aspects of disease*
- Vasodilators and antihypertensives — *to treat Raynaud's phenomenon*
- Digital plaster cast — *to immobilize area, minimize trauma, and maintain cleanliness*
- Possible surgical debridement — *for chronic digital ulceration*
- Antacids and soft, bland diet — *to treat esophagitis*
- Proton pump inhibitors or H2 blockers — *to treat heartburn and protect esophagus and stomach by decreasing stomach acid*
- Vasodilators (short-term benefit) — *to decrease contractility and oxygen demand, and cause vasodilation (for pulmonary hypertension)*
- Physical therapy — *to maintain joint function and promote muscle strength*
- Stress management — to help cope with chronic disease

# Systemic lupus erythematosus

◆ Chronic inflammatory autoimmune disorder of connective tissue
◆ Affects multiple organ systems
◆ Characterized by recurring remissions and exacerbations

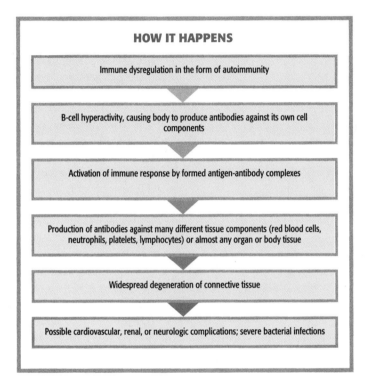

**HOW IT HAPPENS**

Immune dysregulation in the form of autoimmunity

B-cell hyperactivity, causing body to produce antibodies against its own cell components

Activation of immune response by formed antigen-antibody complexes

Production of antibodies against many different tissue components (red blood cells, neutrophils, platelets, lymphocytes) or almost any organ or body tissue

Widespread degeneration of connective tissue

Possible cardiovascular, renal, or neurologic complications; severe bacterial infections

## *Causes*

◆ Unknown
◆ Environmental factors (infections, antibiotics, ultraviolet light, extreme stress, certain drugs, hormones) play critical role in triggering lupus

# ▲ *Pathophysiologic changes*

| | |
|---|---|
| Tissue injury, inflammation, and necrosis from invasion by immune complexes in:<br>– cardiovascular system ➡ | Fever, weight loss, malaise, fatigue, polyarthralgia; cardiac changes (pericarditis, myocarditis, endocarditis, early coronary atherosclerosis); vasculitis (especially in digits), possibly leading to infarctive lesions, necrotic leg ulcers, or digital gangrene; Raynaud's phenomenon |
| – skin and mucous membranes ➡ | Rashes; patchy alopecia and painless ulcers of mucous membranes; skin lesions, notably erythematous rash in areas exposed to light (classic butterfly rash over nose and cheeks occurs in less than half of patients); scaly, papular rash (mimics psoriasis), especially in sun-exposed areas |
| – pulmonary system ➡ | Pulmonary abnormalities (pleurisy, pleural effusions, pneumonitis, pulmonary hypertension) |
| – renal system ➡ | Microscopic hematuria; pyuria; urine sediment with cellular casts |

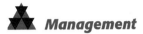 *Management*

- Nonsteroidal anti-inflammatory agents (aspirin) — *to control arthritis symptoms*
- Topical corticosteroid creams (hydrocortisone buteprate or triamcinolone) — *for acute skin lesions*
- Intralesional corticosteroids or antimalarials (hydroxychloroquine sulfate) — *to treat refractory skin lesions*
- Systemic corticosteroids — *to reduce systemic symptoms, for acute generalized exacerbations, or for serious disease related to vital organ systems (pleuritis, pericarditis, lupus nephritis, vasculitis, neurologic involvement)*
- High-dose steroids and cytotoxic therapy (cyclophosphamide [Cytoxan]) — *to treat diffuse proliferative glomerulonephritis*
- Dialysis or kidney transplant — *for renal failure*
- Antihypertensives and dietary changes — to minimize effects of renal involvement

# 8

# Endocrine disorders

## Pathophysiologic concepts   209

## Disorders   210

# PATHOPHYSIOLOGIC CONCEPTS

## *Altered intracellular mechanisms*

◆ Associated with inadequate synthesis of second messenger needed to convert hormonal signal into intracellular events
◆ May involve two different mechanisms
– faulty response of target cells for water-soluble hormones to hormone-receptor binding and failure to generate required second messenger
– abnormal response of target cell to second messenger and failure to express usual hormonal effect

## *Altered receptor mechanisms*

◆ Associated with water-soluble hormones:
– fewer receptors, resulting in diminished or defective hormone-receptor binding
– impaired receptor function, resulting in insensitivity to hormone
– presence of antibodies against specific receptors, either reducing available binding sites or mimicking hormone action and suppressing or exaggerating target cell response

# DISORDERS

## Adrenal hypofunction

♦ Primary hypofunction or insufficiency (Addison's disease) originates within adrenal gland; characterized by decreased secretion of mineralocorticoids, glucocorticoids, and androgens and complete or partial destruction of adrenal cortex

♦ Secondary hypofunction results from disorder outside adrenal gland (impaired pituitary secretion of corticotropin); characterized by decreased glucocorticoid secretion; aldosterone secretion is unaffected

♦ Adrenal crisis (addisonian crisis) involves critical deficiency of mineralocorticoids and glucocorticoids; generally follows acute stress, sepsis, trauma, surgery, or omission of steroid therapy in patients who have chronic adrenal insufficiency

## HOW IT HAPPENS

Acute adrenal crisis, the most serious complication of Addison's disease, involves a critical deficiency of glucocorticoids and mineralocorticoids. This life-threatening event requires prompt assessment and immediate treatment. The flowchart below highlights the underlying mechanisms responsible for it.

Adrenal gland hypofunction

Absent or low cortisol levels

Absent or very low aldosterone levels

**Liver**
Decreased hepatic glucose output

**Stomach**
Reduced levels of digestive enzymes

**Kidneys**
Sodium and water loss with potassium retention

**Heart**
Arrhythmias and decreased cardiac output

Hypoglycemia

Vomiting, cramps, and diarrhea

Hypovolemia          Hypotension

Profound hypoglycemia

Shock

**Brain**
Coma and death

## *Causes*

### *PRIMARY ADRENAL HYPOFUNCTION*
◆ Autoimmune process
◆ Idiopathic atrophy of adrenal glands
◆ Bilateral adrenalectomy
◆ Neoplasms, tuberculosis, or other infections (histoplasmosis, cytomegalovirus, AIDS)

### *SECONDARY ADRENAL HYPOFUNCTION*
◆ Hypopituitarism
◆ Abrupt withdrawal of long-term corticosteroid therapy
◆ Removal of corticotropin-secreting tumor

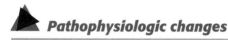

# Pathophysiologic changes

### PRIMARY ADRENAL HYPOFUNCTION

Mineralocorticoid or glucocorticoid deficiency ➤

Weakness, fatigue; weight loss, nausea, vomiting, anorexia; decreased tolerance for even minor stress; cardiovascular abnormalities (orthostatic hypotension; decreased cardiac size and output; weak, irregular pulse), craving for salty food (leads to sodium retention)

Decreased cortisol levels and simultaneous secretion of excessive corticotropin and melanocyte-stimulating hormone ➤

Conspicuous bronze skin coloring, especially in creases of hands and over metacarpophalangeal joints (hand and finger), elbows, and knees; darkening of scars; areas of vitiligo (absence of pigmentation); increased pigmentation of mucous membranes, especially buccal mucosa

Decreased glucogenesis ➤

Fasting hypoglycemia

### SECONDARY ADRENAL HYPOFUNCTION

Low corticotropin and melanocyte-stimulating hormone levels ➤

Signs and symptoms similar to those of primary hypofunction, but without hyperpigmentation

### ACUTE ADRENAL CRISIS

Glucocorticoid and mineralocorticoid deficiencies ➤

Profound weakness and fatigue; nausea and vomiting; dehydration; hypotension; high fever followed by hypothermia (occasionally)

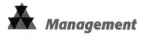 *Management*

♦ Lifelong cortisone or hydrocortisone administration — *for corticosteroid replacement in primary or secondary adrenal hypofunction*
♦ Oral fludrocortisone (Florinef), a synthetic mineralocorticoid — *to prevent dangerous dehydration, hypotension, hyponatremia, and hyperkalemia (Addison's disease)*
♦ I.V. bolus of hydrocortisone (initially for acute adrenal crisis), followed by hydrocortisone diluted with dextrose in I.V. saline solution — *to replace fluids, treat hyponatremia and hypoglycemia, and maintain blood pressure (with proper treatment, adrenal crisis usually subsides quickly; blood pressure stabilizes, and water and sodium levels return to normal)*
♦ Vasopressors (if necessary) — *to treat hypotension uncorrected with initial treatment*
♦ After crisis, maintenance doses of hydrocortisone — *to preserve physiologic stability*

# Cushing's syndrome

◆ Cluster of clinical abnormalities caused by excessive adrenocortical hormones
◆ Cushing's disease (pituitary corticotropin excess) accounts for about 80% of endogenous cases

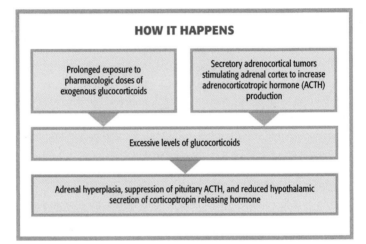

**HOW IT HAPPENS**

Prolonged exposure to pharmacologic doses of exogenous glucocorticoids

Secretory adrenocortical tumors stimulating adrenal cortex to increase adrenocorticotropic hormone (ACTH) production

Excessive levels of glucocorticoids

Adrenal hyperplasia, suppression of pituitary ACTH, and reduced hypothalamic secretion of corticoptropin releasing hormone

## *Causes*

◆ Excess of anterior pituitary hormone (corticotropin)
◆ Ectopic corticotropin secretion by tumor outside pituitary gland
◆ Excessive or prolonged use of glucocorticoids

# ▲ *Pathophysiologic changes*

### ENDOCRINE AND METABOLIC CHANGES

Cortisol-induced insulin resistance and increased gluconeogenesis in liver ➡️

Diabetes mellitus, with decreased glucose tolerance, fasting hyperglycemia, and glucosuria

Increased androgen production ➡️

Mild virilism, hirsutism, clitoral hypertrophy, and amenorrhea or oligomenorrhea (in women); sexual dysfunction

### MUSCULOSKELETAL CHANGES

Hypokalemia ➡️

Muscle weakness

Increased catabolism ➡️

Loss of muscle mass

Decreased bone mineral ionization, osteopenia, osteoporosis, and skeletal growth retardation (in children) ➡️

Pathologic fractures

### SKIN CHANGES

Decreased collagen and weakened tissues ➡️

Purple striae; facial plethora (edema and blood vessel distention); acne; fat pads above clavicles, over upper back (buffalo hump), on face (moon face), and throughout trunk (truncal obesity) with slender arms and legs; little or no scar formation; poor wound healing; spontaneous ecchymosis; hyperpigmentation

### GI CHANGES

Increased gastric secretion and pepsin production ➡️

Peptic ulcer; abdominal pain; increased appetite, weight gain

*(continued)*

## *Pathophysiologic changes (continued)*

### *CARDIOVASCULAR CHANGES*

Sodium and secondary fluid retention ➡ Hypertension, heart failure, left ventricular hypertrophy

Protein loss ➡ Capillary weakness, bleeding, and ecchymosis

### *OTHER CHANGES*

Altered neurotransmission ➡ Irritability and emotional lability

Decreased lymphocyte production and suppressed antibody formation ➡ Increased susceptibility to infection

Increased bone demineralization with hypercalciuria ➡ Fluid retention, increased potassium excretion, ureteral calculi

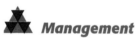 *Management*

- High-potassium, low-sodium, low-carbohydrate, low-calorie, high-protein diet — *to maintain nutritional balance*
- Ketoconazole, metyrapone, and aminoglutethimide — *to inhibit cortisol synthesis*
- Mitotane — *to destroy adrenocortical cells that secrete cortisol*
- Bromocriptine and cyproheptadine — *to inhibit corticotropin secretion*
- Surgical interventions (adrenalectomy, hypophysectomy) — *to control symptoms*
- Radiation therapy (tumor) — *to reduce or eliminate tumor*

# Diabetes mellitus

- Chronic disorder of carbohydrate metabolism with subsequent alteration of protein and fat metabolism
- Characterized by hyperglycemia (elevated serum glucose level) resulting from lack of insulin, lack of insulin effect, or both
- General classifications: type 1 (absolute insulin insufficiency), type 2 (insulin resistance with varying degrees of insulin secretory defects), and gestational diabetes (pregnancy-related)

## THE PATHO PICTURE

### UNDERSTANDING DIABETES MELLITUS

Diabetes affects the way the body uses food to make the energy for life.

#### Type 1 diabetes

- Pancreas makes little or no insulin.
- In genetically susceptible patients, a triggering event (possibly a viral infection) causes production of autoantibodies against the beta cells of the pancreas.
- Resultant destruction of beta cells leads to a decline in and ultimate lack of insulin secretion.
- Insulin deficiency leads to hyperglycemia, enhanced lipolysis, and protein catabolism. These occur when more than 90% of beta cells have been destroyed.

#### Type 2 diabetes

- Genetic factors are significant, and onset is accelerated by obesity and a sedentary lifestyle. The pancreas produces some insulin, but it's either too little or ineffective.
- The following factors contribute to its development:
  – impaired insulin secretion
  – inappropriate hepatic glucose production
  – peripheral insulin receptor insensitivity.

#### Type 1 diabetes

Pancreas with no insulin production

Cell

Glucose

Closed glucose channel

Open glucose channel

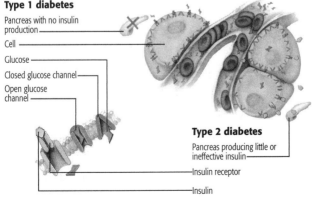

#### Type 2 diabetes

Pancreas producing little or ineffective insulin

Insulin receptor

Insulin

## Causes

### TYPE 1 DIABETES

◆ Autoimmune process triggered by viral or environmental factors
◆ Idiopathic (no evidence of autoimmune process)

### TYPE 2 DIABETES

◆ Beta cell exhaustion due to lifestyle habits or hereditary factors

## Risk factors (type 2 diabetes)

◆ Obesity
◆ Family history
◆ Ethnicity (Black, Hispanic, or Native American)
◆ Women who have given birth to infant weighing more than 9 lb

## ◢ Pathophysiologic changes

| | |
|---|---|
| High serum osmolality caused by high serum glucose levels ➡ | Polyuria, polydipsia |
| Depleted cellular storage of carbohydrate, fat, and protein ➡ | Polyphagia (occasionally in type 1 diabetes) |
| Prevention of normal metabolism of carbohydrate, fat, and protein caused by impaired or absent insulin function ➡ | Weight loss (seen in up to 30% of those with type 1 diabetes; typically patients have almost no body fat at time of diagnosis) |
| Low intracellular glucose levels ➡ | Headache, fatigue, lethargy, reduced energy level |
| Electrolyte imbalances ➡ | Muscle cramps, irritability, and emotional lability |
| Glucose-induced swelling ➡ | Vision changes (blurring) |
| Neural tissue damage ➡ | Numbness and tingling |
| Dehydration, electrolyte imbalances, or autonomic neuropathy ➡ | Abdominal discomfort and pain; nausea, diarrhea, or constipation |
| Hyperglycemia ➡ | Slowly healing skin infections or wounds; skin itching; vaginal pruritus and vulvovaginitis |

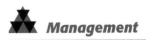

## *Management*

**FOR TYPE 1 DIABETES**

◆ Insulin replacement (mixed-dose, split mixed-dose, and multiple daily injection regimens and continuous subcutaneous insulin infusions), meal planning, and exercise — *to normalize glucose levels and decrease complications*

◆ Pancreas transplantation — *for poorly controlled diabetes to stabilize blood glucose levels and improve quality of life*

**FOR TYPE 2 DIABETES**

◆ Oral antidiabetic drugs — *to stimulate endogenous insulin production, increase insulin sensitivity at cellular level, suppress hepatic gluconeogenesis, and delay GI absorption of carbohydrates*

◆ Insulin therapy (if uncontrolled with oral agents) — *to control blood glucose levels*

**FOR TYPES 1 AND 2 DIABETES**

◆ Careful monitoring of blood glucose levels — *to guide treatment*

◆ Individualized meal plan — *to meet nutritional needs, control blood glucose and lipid levels, and maintain body weight*

◆ Weight reduction (obese patient with type 2 diabetes mellitus) or high-calorie allotment, depending on growth stage and activity level (type 1 diabetes mellitus) — *to ensure adequate nutrition*

◆ Regular, daily physical exercise — *to help control glucose levels*

◆ Patient and family education — *to inform about disease process, potential complications, nutritional management, exercise regimen, blood glucose self-monitoring, insulin and oral medications*

**FOR GESTATIONAL DIABETES**

◆ Nutrition therapy — *to control blood glucose levels*

◆ Insulin (if diet alone is ineffective) — *to control blood glucose levels*

◆ Postpartum counseling — *to address high risk of gestational diabetes in subsequent pregnancies and of type 2 diabetes later*

◆ Regular exercise and prevention of weight gain — *to help prevent type 2 diabetes*

# Hyperthyroidism

◆ Metabolic imbalance that results from overproduction of thyroid hormone; also called thyrotoxicosis

◆ Graves' disease (most common form) increases thyroxine ($T_4$) production, enlarges thyroid gland (goiter), and causes multiple system changes

◆ Thyroid storm (acute, severe exacerbation of thyrotoxicosis), a medical emergency, may have life-threatening cardiac, hepatic, or renal consequences

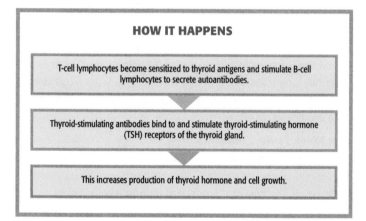

**HOW IT HAPPENS**

T-cell lymphocytes become sensitized to thyroid antigens and stimulate B-cell lymphocytes to secrete autoantibodies.

Thyroid-stimulating antibodies bind to and stimulate thyroid-stimulating hormone (TSH) receptors of the thyroid gland.

This increases production of thyroid hormone and cell growth.

## Causes

◆ Autoimmune disease (Graves' disease)
◆ Genetic factors
◆ Thyroid adenomas
◆ Toxic multinodular goiter
◆ Increased thyroid-stimulating hormone (TSH) secretions
◆ Precipitating factors (infection, surgery, toxemia of pregnancy, diabetic ketoacidosis, stress)

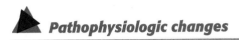 *Pathophysiologic changes*

**HYPERTHYROIDISM**

Increased amounts of thyroid hormone ➡

Enlarged thyroid (goiter); excitability or nervousness; heat intolerance and sweating; weight loss (despite increased appetite); frequent bowel movements; palpitations; hypertension

Cytokine-mediated activation of orbital tissue fibroblasts ➡

Exophthalmos

Accelerated cerebral function ➡

Difficulty concentrating

Increased activity in spinal cord area that controls muscle tone ➡

Fine tremor, shaky handwriting, clumsiness

**THYROID STORM**

Increased catecholamine response and hyperthyroid state

High fever, tachycardia, pulmonary edema, hypertension, shock, tremors, emotional lability, extreme irritability, confusion, delirium, psychosis, apathy, stupor, coma, diarrhea, abdominal pain, nausea, vomiting, jaundice, hyperglycemia

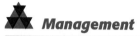 *Management*

♦ Antithyroid drugs — *to treat new-onset Graves' disease (spontaneous remission possible) and to correct thyrotoxic state in preparation for radioactive iodine ($^{131}I$) treatment or surgery*

♦ Thyroid hormone antagonists, including propylthiouracil (PTU) and methimazole (Tapazole) — *to block thyroid hormone synthesis*

♦ Beta-adrenergic blocker (propranolol [Inderal]) until antithyroid drugs reach their full effect — *to manage tachycardia and other peripheral effects of excessive hypersympathetic activity*

♦ Iodine preparations (potassium iodine, $^{131}I$) — *to decrease thyroid gland's capacity for hormone production*

♦ Subtotal thyroidectomy (for those who refuse or aren't candidates for $^{131}I$ treatment) — *to decrease thyroid gland's capacity for hormone production*

♦ Lifelong, regular medical supervision — *to treat hypothyroidism, which develops in most patients after surgery (sometimes several years later)*

# Hypothyroidism, adult

◆ Results from hypothalamic, pituitary, or thyroid insufficiency or resistance to thyroid hormone
◆ Can progress to life-threatening myxedema coma

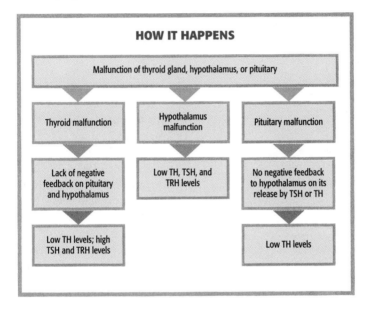

*Causes*

◆ Autoimmune disease (Hashimoto's thyroiditis)
◆ Overuse of antithyroid drugs
◆ Thyroidectomy
◆ Malfunction of pituitary gland
◆ Radiation therapy (particularly with iodine 131 [[131]I])

# ▲ *Pathophysiologic changes*

| | |
|---|---|
| Hypometabolic state ▶ | Weakness, fatigue, forgetfulness, delayed deep tendon reflexes, sensitivity to cold, unexplained weight gain, constipation, menorrhagia, decreased libido, and infertility |
| Fluid accumulation ▶ | Characteristic signs and symptoms of myxedema:<br>– puffy face, hands, and feet<br>– hoarseness<br>– periorbital edema<br>– upper eyelid droop<br>– dry, sparse hair; thick, brittle nails; rough, dry skin with yellowish appearance (as disorder progresses due to carotene deposition) |
| Cardiovascular involvement related to mucopolysaccharide deposits ▶ | Decreased cardiac output, slow pulse rate, signs of poor peripheral circulation, enlarged heart (occasionally) |
| Progression to myxedema coma (usually gradual but may occur abruptly; related to stress-aggravating severe or prolonged hypothyroidism) ▶ | Progressive stupor, hypoventilation, hypoglycemia, hyponatremia, hypotension, hypothermia |

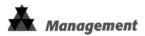

# Management

- ◆ Gradual thyroid hormone replacement (with synthetic T$_4$ and, occasionally, T$_3$) — *to replace needed hormones*
- ◆ High-bulk, low-calorie diet — *to maintain adequate nutritional status*
- ◆ Cathartics and stool softeners (as needed) — *to maintain bowel function*
- ◆ Surgical excision, chemotherapy, or radiation (for tumors) — *to reduce size of or remove tumor*

# Syndrome of inappropriate antidiuretic hormone (SIADH)

◆ Potentially life-threatening condition that disturbs fluid and electrolyte balance
◆ Results when excessive antidiuretic hormone (ADH) secretion is triggered by stimuli other than increased extracellular fluid osmolarity and decreased extracellular fluid volume, reflected by hypotension

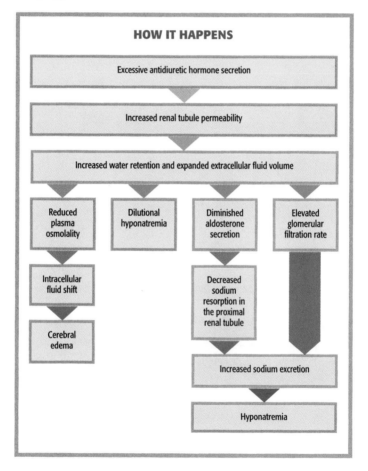

**HOW IT HAPPENS**

Excessive antidiuretic hormone secretion

↓

Increased renal tubule permeability

↓

Increased water retention and expanded extracellular fluid volume

| Reduced plasma osmolality | Dilutional hyponatremia | Diminished aldosterone secretion | Elevated glomerular filtration rate |

Intracellular fluid shift

Decreased sodium resorption in the proximal renal tubule

Cerebral edema

Increased sodium excretion

Hyponatremia

## *Causes*

◆ Oat cell carcinoma of lung (most common cause; secretes excessive levels of ADH or vasopressin-like substances)
◆ Neoplastic diseases (pancreatic or prostate cancer, Hodgkin's disease, thymoma, renal carcinoma)
◆ Less common causes:
   – central nervous system disorders (brain tumor or abscess, stroke, head injury, Guillain-Barré syndrome)
   – pulmonary disorders (pneumonia, tuberculosis, lung abscess, aspergillosis, bronchiectasis, positive-pressure ventilation)
   – drugs that either increase ADH production or potentiate ADH action (antidepressants, nonsteroidal anti-inflammatory drugs, chlorpropamide [Diabinese], vincristine [Oncovin], cyclophosphamide [Cytoxan], carbamazepine [Tegretol], clofibrate [Atromid-S], metoclopramide [Reglan], morphine)
   – miscellaneous conditions (psychosis, myxedema, acquired immunodeficiency syndrome, physiologic stress, pain)

## ◢ *Pathophysiologic changes*

| | |
|---|---|
| Hyponatremia and electrolyte imbalances ➡ | Thirst, anorexia, fatigue, and lethargy (first signs), followed by vomiting and intestinal cramping; weight gain, edema, water retention, and decreased urine output; neurologic changes (restlessness, confusion, headache, irritability, decreasing reflexes, and seizures); coma; decreased deep tendon reflexes |

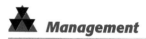 *Management*

◆ Restricted water intake (500 to 1,000 ml/day) — *to treat symptoms*

◆ Administration of 200 to 300 ml of 3% saline solution — *to slowly and steadily increase serum sodium level (severe water intoxication); if too rapid a rise, cerebral edema may result*

◆ Correction of underlying cause (when possible) — *to relieve symptoms*

◆ Surgical resection, irradiation, or chemotherapy — *to alleviate water retention for SIADH resulting from cancer*

◆ Demeclocycline (Declomycin) — *to block renal response to ADH (if fluid restriction is ineffective)*

◆ Furosemide (Lasix) with normal or hypertonic saline — *to maintain urine output and block ADH secretion*

# 9

# Renal disorders

# PATHOPHYSIOLOGIC CONCEPTS

## *Altered capillary pressure*

◆ Capillary pressure reflects mean arterial pressure (MAP)
  – Increased MAP increases capillary pressure and glomerular filtration rate (GFR)
  – Decreased MAP lowers capillary pressure and GFR
  – GFR decreases steeply if MAP decreases to < 80 mm Hg
◆ Autoregulation of afferent and efferent arterioles affects capillary pressure
  – Increased sympathetic activity and angiotensin II constrict afferent and efferent arterioles, decreasing capillary pressure
  – Prostaglandin-mediated relaxation of afferent arterioles and angiotensin II–mediated constriction of efferent arterioles maintain GFR
◆ Decreased cardiac output diminishes renal perfusion (inadequate renal perfusion accounts for 40% to 80% of acute renal failure)
  – Hypovolemia may reduce circulating blood volume and decreases MAP
  – Prolonged renal hypoperfusion causes acute tubular necrosis
◆ Drugs that block prostaglandin production (NSAIDs) can cause vasoconstriction and acute renal failure during hypotension
◆ Emboli or thrombi, aortic dissection, or vasculitis can occlude renal arteries

## *Altered interstitial fluid colloid osmotic pressure*

◆ Injury to glomeruli or peritubular capillaries can increase interstitial fluid colloid osmotic pressure, drawing fluid out of glomerulus and peritubular capillaries
  – Swelling and edema occur in Bowman's space and interstitial space surrounding tubule
  – Increased interstitial fluid pressure opposes glomerular filtration, causes collapse of surrounding nephrons and peritubular capillaries, and leads to hypoxia and renal cell injury or death
  – When cells die, intracellular enzymes are released, stimulating immune and inflammatory reactions
  – Increased interstitial fluid pressure interferes with glomerular filtration and tubular resorption; renders kidney incapable of regulating blood volume and electrolyte composition
◆ Glomerular disease disrupts basement membrane, allowing leakage of large proteins
  – Plasma oncotic pressure decreases and edema results as fluid moves from capillaries into interstitium
  – Consequent activation of renin-angiotensin system and sympathetic nervous system increases renal salt and water resorption, which further contributes to edema

## *Obstruction*

◆ Causes urine to accumulate behind blockage in urinary tract, leading to infection or damage
◆ May be congenital or acquired, acute or chronic
  – acute, complete obstruction increases pressure transmitted to proximal tubule, inhibiting glomerular filtration
  – chronic, partial obstruction compresses structures as urine accumulates; results in papillary and medullary infarct; underlying tubular damage decreases kidney's ability to function
◆ Tubular obstruction increases interstitial fluid pressure; if unrelieved, causes nephron and capillary collapse and irreversible renal damage
◆ Relief is usually followed by copious diuresis of sodium and water and return to normal GFR

# DISORDERS

## Acute renal failure

- Sudden interruption of renal function caused by obstruction, poor circulation, or underlying kidney disease
- Classified as prerenal, intrarenal, or postrenal
- Involves three distinct phases: oliguric, diuretic, and recovery
- Usually reversible with treatment; untreated may progress to end-stage renal disease, prerenal azotemia, and death

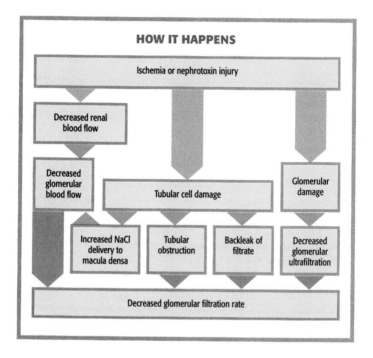

**HOW IT HAPPENS**

Ischemia or nephrotoxin injury

Decreased renal blood flow

Decreased glomerular blood flow

Tubular cell damage

Glomerular damage

Increased NaCl delivery to macula densa

Tubular obstruction

Backleak of filtrate

Decreased glomerular ultrafiltration

Decreased glomerular filtration rate

## *Causes*

### *PRERENAL FAILURE*
◆ Arrhythmias, cardiac tamponade, cardiogenic shock, heart failure, myocardial infarction
◆ Burns, trauma, sepsis
◆ Dehydration, hypovolemic shock
◆ Diuretic overuse, antihypertensive drugs
◆ Hemorrhage, arterial embolism, arterial or venous thrombosis, vasculitis
◆ Disseminated intravascular coagulation
◆ Eclampsia, malignant hypertension

### *INTRARENAL FAILURE*
◆ Poorly treated prerenal failure
◆ Nephrotoxins
◆ Obstetric complications
◆ Crush injuries, myopathy
◆ Transfusion reaction
◆ Acute glomerulonephritis, acute interstitial nephritis, acute pyelonephritis, bilateral renal vein thrombosis
◆ Malignant nephrosclerosis
◆ Sickle cell disease
◆ Systemic lupus erythematosus
◆ Vasculitis

### *POSTRENAL FAILURE*
◆ Bladder obstruction, ureteral obstruction, urethral obstruction

## ▲ *Pathophysiologic changes*

| | |
|---|---|
| Decreased blood flow ➤ | Early signs: Oliguria, azotemia, anuria (rarely) |
| Increasing uremia and renal dysfunction ➤ | Electrolyte imbalance, metabolic acidosis |
| Electrolyte imbalance ➤ | Anorexia, nausea, vomiting, diarrhea |
| Altered cerebral perfusion ➤ | Headache, drowsiness, irritability, confusion, peripheral neuropathy, seizures, coma |
| Buildup of toxins and stimulation of sympathetic nervous system ➤ | Dry skin, pruritus, pallor, purpura, dry mucous membranes, uremic frost (rare) |
| Altered volume status ➤ | Hypotension (early), hypertension (later), arrhythmias, fluid overload, heart failure, systemic edema, anemia, altered clotting mechanisms |

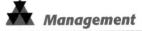 *Management*

◆ High-calorie diet that is low in protein, sodium, and potassium — *to meet metabolic needs*
◆ Careful monitoring of electrolytes, I.V. therapy — *to maintain and correct fluid and electrolyte balance*
◆ Fluid restriction — *to minimize edema*
◆ Diuretic therapy — *to treat oliguric phase*
◆ Low-dose dopamine — *to enhance renal perfusion*
◆ Atrial natriuretic peptide — *to improve perfusion to glomeruli by inhibiting sodium and water absorption and dilating afferent arteriole*
◆ Sodium polystyrene sulfonate (Kayexalate) by mouth or enema — *to reverse hyperkalemia with mild hyperkalemic symptoms (malaise, loss of appetite, muscle weakness)*
◆ Hypertonic glucose, insulin, and sodium bicarbonate I.V. — *for more severe hyperkalemic symptoms (numbness, tingling, ECG changes)*
◆ Hemodialysis, continuous renal replacement therapy, or peritoneal dialysis — *to correct electrolyte and fluid imbalances*

# Acute tubular necrosis

◆ Most common cause of acute renal failure; also known as acute tubulointerstitial nephritis
◆ Results from ischemia or nephrotoxicity
  – Ischemic injury (most common) interrupts blood flow to kidneys
  – Nephrotoxic injury usually affects debilitated patients (critically ill and those who have undergone extensive surgery)
◆ Causes injury to nephron's tubular segment; may lead to renal failure and uremic syndrome

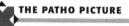
**THE PATHO PICTURE**

## UNDERSTANDING ACUTE TUBULAR NECROSIS

Acute tubular necrosis results from ischemia or nephrotoxic injury. When caused by ischemia, necrosis typically develops as patches in straight portions of the proximal tubules, creating deep lesions that destroy the tubular epithelium and basement membrane. In areas without lesions, tubules usually are dilated.

Ischemic damage

With nephrotoxic injury, necrosis occurs only in the epithelium of the tubules, leaving the basement membrane of the nephrons intact; consequently, the damage may be reversible. The tubules maintain a more uniform appearance.

Toxic damage

## *Causes*

### *ISCHEMIC INJURY*
◆ Circulatory collapse, severe hypotension
◆ Trauma, hemorrhage, severe dehydration
◆ Cardiogenic or septic shock
◆ Surgery, anesthetics, or transfusion reactions

### *NEPHROTOXIC INJURY*
◆ Ingesting or inhaling toxic chemicals
◆ Hypersensitivity reaction of kidneys to antibiotics, radiographic contrast agents

## ◢ *Pathophysiologic changes*

| | |
|---|---|
| Marked decrease in glomerular filtration rate ➡ | Common signs and symptoms (may be masked by critically ill patient's primary disease): <br> – Decreased urine output (generally first recognizable effect) <br> – Hyperkalemia (with characteristic ECG changes) <br> – Elevated serum creatinine and BUN levels <br> – Dry mucous membranes and skin <br> – CNS changes: lethargy, twitching, or seizures <br> – Uremic syndrome: oliguria or anuria (rare) and confusion, which may progress to uremic coma; oliguric phase may not be present in some patients because of higher levels of glomerular filtration |
| Return of BUN and creatinine levels to normal (recovery phase) ➡ | Diuresis |

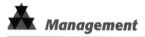 *Management*

### FOR ACUTE PHASE

◆ Vigorous supportive measures until normal kidney function resumes — *to prevent further injury to kidney*
◆ Initially, possible administration of diuretics and infusion of large volume of fluids — *to flush tubules of cellular casts and debris and to replace fluid loss (risk of fluid overload with this treatment)*

### FOR LONG-TERM FLUID MANAGEMENT

◆ Daily replacement of projected and calculated losses (including insensible loss) — *to maintain fluid balance*

### FOR PREVENTION OF COMPLICATIONS

◆ Transfusion of packed red blood cells — *for anemia*
◆ Administration of antibiotics — *for infection*
◆ Emergency I.V. administration of 50% glucose, regular insulin, and sodium bicarbonate — *for hyperkalemia*
◆ Sodium polystyrene sulfonate with sorbitol by mouth or enema — *to reduce extracellular potassium levels*
◆ Peritoneal dialysis, hemodialysis, or continuous renal replacement therapy — *to prevent severe fluid and electrolyte imbalance and uremia*

# Bladder cancer

◆ May develop on surface of bladder wall (benign or malignant papillomas) or grow within bladder wall (generally more virulent) and quickly invade underlying muscles
◆ Most common type: transitional cell carcinoma, arising from transitional epithelium of mucous membranes
◆ Less common types: adenocarcinomas, epidermoid carcinomas, squamous cell carcinomas, sarcomas, tumors in bladder diverticula, and carcinoma in situ
◆ Early stages commonly asymptomatic

**THE PATHO PICTURE**

### HOW BLADDER CANCER DEVELOPS

Bladder tumors can develop on the surface of the bladder wall or grow within the bladder wall and quickly invade underlying muscle. Most bladder tumors (90%) are transitional cell carcinomas, arising from the transitional epithelium of mucous membranes. They also may result from malignant transformation of benign papillomas. The illustration below shows a bladder carcinoma infiltrating the bladder wall.

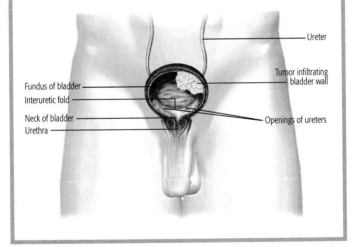

Ureter

Tumor infiltrating bladder wall

Fundus of bladder
Interuretic fold

Neck of bladder
Urethra

Openings of ureters

## *Cause*

◆ Primary cause unknown

## *Risk factors*

◆ Environmental carcinogens (2-naphthylamine, tobacco, nitrates)
◆ Schistosomiasis (squamous cell carcinoma of bladder; most common in endemic areas)
◆ Chronic bladder irritation and infection

### ▲ *Pathophysiologic changes*

| | |
|---|---|
| Tumor invasion ➡ | **Gross, painless, intermittent hematuria** |
| Pressure exerted by tumor or obstruction ➡ | **Suprapubic pain after voiding** |
| Tumor compression and invasion ➡ | **Bladder irritability, urinary frequency, nocturia, and dribbling** |

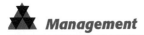 *Management*

### FOR SUPERFICIAL BLADDER TUMORS

◆ Transurethral (cystoscopic) resection and fulguration (electrical destruction) — *to remove tumor*
◆ Intravesicular chemotherapy (for multiple tumors) — *to kill cancer cells*
◆ Fulguration if additional tumors develop (may be repeated every 3 months for years) — *to remove tumor*

### FOR LARGE TUMOR

◆ Segmental bladder resection — *to remove full-thickness section of bladder (only if tumor isn't near bladder neck or ureteral orifices)*
◆ Bladder instillations of thiotepa after transurethral resection — *to slow or stop growth of cancer cells*

### FOR INFILTRATING BLADDER TUMORS

◆ Radical cystectomy — *treatment of choice for infiltrating bladder tumors (requires urinary diversion, usually ileal conduit)*
◆ Possible penile implant (later) — *to treat erectile dysfunction*
◆ Referral to American Cancer Society, United Ostomy Association (if patient received ostomy) — *for information and support*

### ADVANCED BLADDER CANCER

◆ Cystectomy — *to remove tumor*
◆ Radiation therapy — *to destroy cancer cells*
◆ Systemic chemotherapy (cisplatin, cyclophosphamide, fluorouracil, doxorubicin) — *to destroy cancer cells*
◆ Investigational treatments (clinical trials currently being conducted):
  – photodynamic therapy and intravesicular administration of interferon alfa and tumor necrosis factor — *to destroy cancer cells*
  – BCG (immunomodulating agent) — *to treat superficial bladder cancer after surgery to remove tumor*
  – biologic response modifiers (interferons, interleukins, colony-stimulating factors, monoclonal antibodies, vaccines) — *to destroy cancer cells*

# Chronic renal failure

- ◆ Usually, end result of gradual tissue destruction and loss of renal function
- ◆ May also result from rapidly progressing disease of sudden onset that destroys nephrons and causes irreversible kidney damage
- ◆ Few symptoms until less than 25% of glomerular filtration remains; normal parenchyma then deteriorates rapidly, and symptoms worsen as renal function decreases
- ◆ Fatal without treatment; dialysis or kidney transplant can sustain life

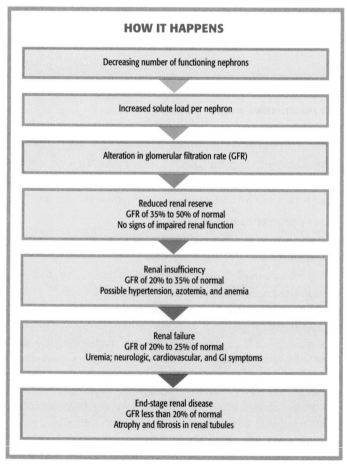

**HOW IT HAPPENS**

Decreasing number of functioning nephrons

Increased solute load per nephron

Alteration in glomerular filtration rate (GFR)

Reduced renal reserve
GFR of 35% to 50% of normal
No signs of impaired renal function

Renal insufficiency
GFR of 20% to 35% of normal
Possible hypertension, azotemia, and anemia

Renal failure
GFR of 20% to 25% of normal
Uremia; neurologic, cardiovascular, and GI symptoms

End-stage renal disease
GFR less than 20% of normal
Atrophy and fibrosis in renal tubules

## *Causes*

- ◆ Chronic glomerular disease (glomerulonephritis)
- ◆ Chronic infection (chronic pyelonephritis and tuberculosis)
- ◆ Congenital anomalies (polycystic kidney disease)
- ◆ Vascular disease (hypertension, nephrosclerosis)
- ◆ Obstruction (renal calculi)
- ◆ Collagen disease (lupus erythematosus)
- ◆ Nephrotoxic agents (long-term aminoglycoside therapy)
- ◆ Endocrine disease (diabetic neuropathy)

## *Pathophysiologic changes*

| | |
|---|---|
| Fluid and electrolyte imbalance ▶ | Hypervolemia, hypocalcemia, hyperkalemia; dry mouth, fatigue, nausea; altered mental state; irregular heart rate and cardiac irritability; muscle cramps and twitching; hypertension |
| Loss of bicarbonate ▶ | Kussmaul's respirations, metabolic acidosis |
| Calcium-phosphorus imbalance and consequent parathyroid hormone imbalances ▶ | Bone and muscle pain and fractures |
| Accumulation of toxins ▶ | Pain, burning (itching in legs and feet), peripheral neuropathy |
| Altered metabolic processes ▶ | Yellow-bronze skin; dry, scaly skin and severe itching; azotemia |
| Endocrine disturbances ▶ | Infertility; decreased libido, amenorrhea, impotence |
| Thrombocytopenia and platelet defects ▶ | GI bleeding, hemorrhage, bruising; gum soreness and bleeding |
| Decreased macrophage activity ▶ | Susceptibility to infection |

*Management*

♦ Low-protein diet — *to limit accumulation of end products of protein metabolism that kidneys can't excrete*

♦ Sodium, potassium, and fluid restrictions — *to maintain fluid and electrolyte balance*

♦ Loop diuretics (furosemide [Lasix]) — *to maintain fluid balance*

♦ Cardiac glycosides (digoxin) — *to mobilize fluids causing edema*

♦ Calcium carbonate (Caltrate) or calcium acetate (PhosLo) — *to treat renal osteodystrophy by binding phosphate and supplementing calcium*

♦ Antihypertensives (ACE inhibitors) — *to control blood pressure and edema*

♦ Famotidine (Pepcid) or ranitidine (Zantac) — *to decrease gastric irritation*

♦ Iron and folate supplements or RBC transfusion — *for anemia*

♦ Synthetic erythropoietin — *to stimulate bone marrow to produce RBCs*

♦ Supplemental iron, conjugated estrogens, and desmopressin — *to combat hematologic effects*

♦ Peritoneal dialysis or hemodialysis — *to treat fluid imbalance and help control end-stage renal disease*

♦ Renal transplantation (usually treatment of choice if donor is available) — *to replace patient's malfunctioning kidneys*

# Glomerulonephritis

◆ Bilateral inflammation of glomeruli; may be acute or chronic
  – Acute form (also called acute poststreptococcal glomerulonephritis) typically follows streptococcal infection
  – Chronic form is characterized by inflammation, sclerosis,
  scarring and, eventually, renal failure; typically remains unde-
  tected until progressive phase (usually irreversible)
◆ Rapidly progressive glomerulonephritis (RPGN) — subacute,
  crescentic, or extracapillary glomerulonephritis — may be idiopathic or associated with proliferative glomerular disease
◆ Goodpasture's syndrome (type of rapidly progressive glomerulonephritis) is rare

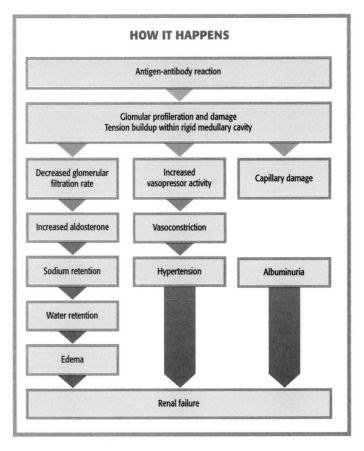

**HOW IT HAPPENS**

Antigen-antibody reaction

Glomular profileration and damage
Tension buildup within rigid medullary cavity

| Decreased glomerular filtration rate | Increased vasopressor activity | Capillary damage |
| Increased aldosterone | Vasoconstriction | |
| Sodium retention | Hypertension | Albuminuria |
| Water retention | | |
| Edema | | |

Renal failure

## *Causes*

### *ACUTE GLOMERULONEPHRITIS AND RPGN*
♦ Streptococcal infection of respiratory tract
♦ Impetigo
♦ Immunoglobulin (Ig) A nephropathy (Berger's disease)
♦ Lipoid nephrosis

### *CHRONIC GLOMERULONEPHRITIS*
♦ Membranoproliferative glomerulonephritis
♦ Membranous glomerulopathy
♦ Focal glomerulosclerosis
♦ RPGN
♦ Poststreptococcal glomerulonephritis
♦ Systemic lupus erythematosus
♦ Goodpasture's syndrome
♦ Hemolytic uremic syndrome

## *Pathophysiologic changes*

| | |
|---|---|
| Decreased glomerular filtration rate (GFR) ➡ | **Decreased urination or oliguria** |
| Hematuria ➡ | **Smoky or coffee-colored urine** |
| Hypervolemia ➡ | **Dyspnea and orthopnea; periorbital edema; bi-basilar crackles** |
| Decreased GFR, sodium or water retention, and inappropriate release of rennin ➡ | **Mild to severe hypertension** |

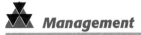

## Management

- Treatment of primary disease — *to alter immunologic cascade*
- Antibiotics for 7 to 10 days — *to treat infections contributing to ongoing antigen-antibody response*
- Anticoagulants — *to control fibrin crescent formation in RPGN*
- Bed rest — *to reduce metabolic demands*
- Fluid restrictions — *to decrease edema*
- Dietary sodium restriction — *to prevent fluid retention*
- Loop diuretics (metolazone [Zaroxolyn] or furosemide [Lasix]) — *to reduce extracellular fluid overload*
- Vasodilators (hydralazine [Apresoline] or nifedipine [Procardia]) — *to decrease hypertension*
- Corticosteroids — *to decrease antibody synthesis and suppress inflammatory response*
- Plasmapheresis (in RPGN), possibly combined with corticosteroids and cyclophosphamide (Cytoxin) — *to suppress rebound antibody production*
- Dialysis (for chronic glomerulonephritis) — *to correct fluid and electrolyte imbalances*
- Kidney transplantation — *to replace patient's malfunctioning kidneys*

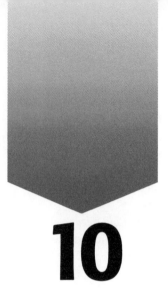

# 10

# Integumentary disorders

# PATHOPHYSIOLOGIC CONCEPTS

## *Lesion formation*

◆ Primary lesions appear on previously healthy skin in response to disease or external irritation
◆ Primary lesion classifications: macules, papules, plaques, patches, nodules, tumors, wheals, comedos, cysts, vesicles, pustules, or bullae
◆ Modified lesions are secondary skin lesions
  – Result from rupture, mechanical irritation, extension, invasion, or normal or abnormal healing of primary lesions
  – Classified as atrophy, erosions, ulcers, scales, crusts, excoriation, fissures, lichenification, and scars

## *Skin inflammation*

◆ Reaction of vascularized tissue to injury
◆ Skin changes caused by inflammatory response
◆ Increased immunoglobulin E activity resulting from immune response to infectious organism, trauma, extreme heat or cold, chemical irritation, or ischemic changes

# DISORDERS

## Basal cell carcinoma

◆ Slow-growing, destructive skin tumor; also called basal cell epithelioma
◆ Accounts for more than 50% of all cancers
◆ Changes in epidermal basal cells can diminish maturation and normal keratinization; continuing division of basal cells leads to mass formation

**THE PATHO PICTURE**

### HOW BASAL CELL CARCINOMA DEVELOPS

Basal cell carcinoma is thought to originate when undifferentiated basal cells become carcinomatous instead of differentiating into sweat glands, sebum, and hair. The most common cancer, it begins as a papule, enlarges, and develops a central crater. Usually, this cancer spreads only locally.

### Causes

◆ Prolonged sun exposure (most common)
◆ Arsenic, radiation exposure, burns, immunosuppression, vaccinations (rare)

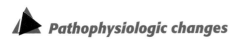

# Pathophysiologic changes

### NODULO-ULCERATIVE LESIONS

Unrepaired mutations in skin cells ➡

Appear most commonly on face (forehead, eyelid margins, nasolabial folds)
– Early stages: lesions are small, smooth, pinkish, translucent papules; telangiectatic vessels cross surface, lesions are occasionally pigmented
– As lesions enlarge: depressed center with firm, elevated borders
– Ulceration and local invasion: rodent ulcers (chronic, persisting ulcers that spread locally) eventually occur but rarely metastasize; untreated can spread to vital areas and become infected; may cause massive hemorrhage if invasion of large blood vessels occurs

### SUPERFICIAL BASAL CELL CARCINOMA

Unrepaired mutations in skin cells ➡

Often numerous and commonly occur on chest and back
– Oval or irregularly shaped, lightly pigmented plaques, with sharply defined, slightly elevated threadlike borders
– Superficial erosion: lesions appear scaly and have small, atrophic areas in center, resembling psoriasis or eczema

### SCLEROSING BASAL CELL CARCINOMA (MORPHEA-LIKE EPITHELIOMAS)

Unrepaired mutations in skin cells ➡

Occur on head and neck
– Lesions appear waxy, sclerotic, yellow to white plaques, without distinct borders

# ▲▲ *Management*

- ◆ Curettage and electrodesiccation — *to remove small lesions (offers good cosmetic results)*
- ◆ Topical fluorouracil — *to treat superficial lesions (produces marked local irritation or inflammation but no systemic effects)*
- ◆ Microscopically controlled surgical excision — *to carefully remove recurrent lesions until tumor-free plane is achieved (after removal of large lesions, skin grafting may be required)*
- ◆ Irradiation (use depends on tumor location and if patient is elderly or debilitated and unable to withstand surgery) — *to eradicate tumor*
- ◆ Cryotherapy (with liquid nitrogen) — *to freeze and kill cancerous cells*
- ◆ Chemosurgery (may be necessary for persistent or recurrent lesions) — *to kill cancer cells*

# Cellulitis

◆ Infection of dermis or subcutaneous layer of skin, possibly resulting from skin damage (bite or wound)
◆ May cause fever, erythema, or lymphangitis
◆ Risk factors: diabetes, immunodeficiency, impaired circulation, neuropathy

**THE PATHO PICTURE**

### UNDERSTANDING CELLULITIS

An acute, spreading infection of the dermis or subcutaneous layer of the skin, cellulitis may result from damage to the skin, such as a bite or wound. The offending organism invades the compromised area and overwhelms the normal defensive cells (neutrophils, eosinophils, basophils, and mast cells) that normally contain and localize inflammation, causing cellular debris to accumulate. As cellulitis progresses, the organism invades surrounding tissue around the initial wound.

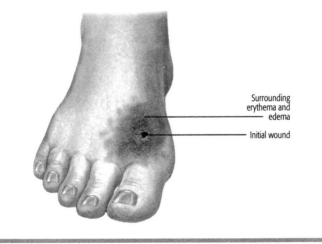

Surrounding erythema and edema

Initial wound

## Causes

◆ Bacterial and fungal infections, commonly group A streptococcus and *Staphylococcus aureus*
◆ Sepsis (in infants), usually group B streptococci

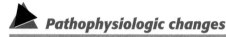 *Pathophysiologic changes*

| Inflammatory response to injury 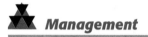 | Erythema and edema; pain at site of infection and possibly surrounding area; fever; lymphadenitis |

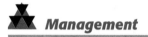 *Management*

- ◆ Oral or I.V. penicillin (drug of choice for initial treatment unless patient is allergic) — *to treat infection*
- ◆ Warm soaks to site — *to increase vasodilation*
- ◆ Analgesics — *to treat pain*
- ◆ Elevation of infected extremity — *to promote comfort and decrease edema*
- ◆ Protective footwear — *for ambulation*

# Contact dermatitis

◆ Sharply demarcated inflammation of skin
◆ Results from contact with irritating chemical or atopic allergen
◆ Produces varying symptoms, depending on type and degree of exposure

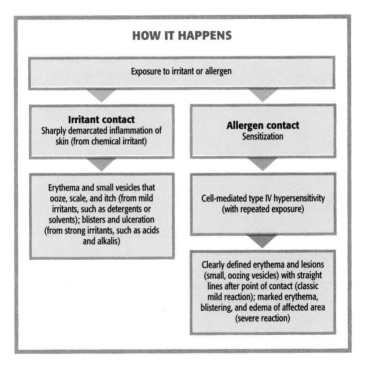

## *Causes*

◆ Mild irritants: chronic exposure to detergents or solvents
◆ Strong irritants: damage or contact with acids or alkalis
◆ Allergens: sensitization after repeated exposure

# ▲ *Pathophysiologic changes*

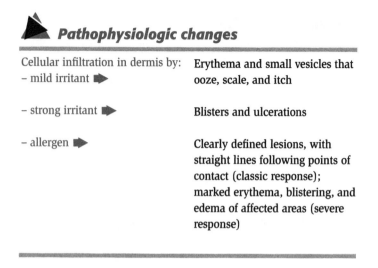

| Cellular infiltration in dermis by: | |
|---|---|
| – mild irritant ➡ | Erythema and small vesicles that ooze, scale, and itch |
| – strong irritant ➡ | Blisters and ulcerations |
| – allergen ➡ | Clearly defined lesions, with straight lines following points of contact (classic response); marked erythema, blistering, and edema of affected areas (severe response) |

# ▲ *Management*

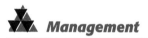

◆ Elimination of known allergens, decreased exposure to irritants, wearing protective clothing (gloves), washing immediately after contact with irritants or allergens — *to prevent reaction*
◆ Topical anti-inflammatory agents (including corticosteroids), antihistamines, and systemic corticosteroids — *for edema and bullae*

# Herpes zoster

◆ Acute inflammation caused by infection with herpesvirus varicella-zoster (chickenpox virus); also called shingles
◆ Produces localized vesicular skin lesions and severe neuralgic pain in peripheral areas
◆ Most patients (usually occurs in adults) recover completely, but may cause scarring, visual impairment (with corneal damage), or persistent neuralgia

**THE PATHO PICTURE**

### UNDERSTANDING HERPES ZOSTER

Herpes zoster erupts when the varicella-zoster virus reactivates after dormancy in the ganglia of the posterior nerve roots or in the cerebral ganglia (extramedullary ganglia of the cranial nerves). The virus may multiply as it reactivates, and antibodies remaining from the initial infection may neutralize it. However, without opposition from effective antibodies, the virus will continue to multiply in the ganglia, destroying neurons and spreading down the sensory nerves to the skin.

The classic vesicles of herpes zoster (shown here) have erupted along a peripheral nerve in the torso.

This illustration shows the lesions about 10 days later – after they've begun to dry and form scabs.

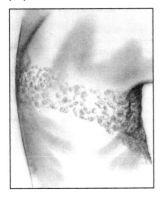
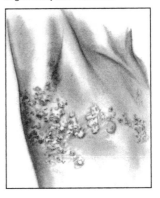

## *Cause*

◆ Reactivation of varicella virus

## ▲ *Pathophysiologic changes*

| | |
|---|---|
| Viral reactivation ▶ | Fever and malaise; eruption of small, red, nodular skin lesions on painful areas<br>– Lesions commonly spread unilaterally around thorax or vertically over arms or legs<br>– Nodules (sometimes none appear) quickly become vesicles filled with clear fluid or pus |
| Innervation of nerves arising in inflamed root ganglia ▶ | Severe deep pain, pruritus, and paresthesia or hyperesthesia<br>– Usually develop on trunk; occasionally on arms and legs in dermatomal distribution<br>– Pain may be continuous or intermittent; usually lasts 1 to 4 weeks |
| Trigeminal ganglion involvement ▶ | Eye pain, corneal and scleral damage (possible), impaired vision |
| Oculomotor involvement (rare) ▶ | Conjunctivitis, extraocular weakness, ptosis, paralytic mydriasis |

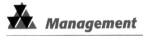 *Management*

- Antiviral agent (acyclovir, treatment of choice) — *to help stop rash progression, prevent visceral complications, and shorten duration of pain and symptoms in normal adults; may be given I.V. to prevent life-threatening disease in immunocompromised patients*
- Use of calamine lotion (or another antipruritic) and analgesics (aspirin, acetaminophen, codeine) — *to relieve itching and neuralgic pain*
- Systemic antibiotic — *to treat bacterial-infected ruptured vesicles*
- Immediate follow-up with ophthalmologist and instillation of idoxuridine ointment (or another antiviral agent) — *to treat trigeminal zoster with corneal involvement*
- Corticosteroid (cortisone) or possibly tricyclic antidepressants, anticonvulsant agents, or nerve block — *to reduce inflammation and help patient cope with intractable pain of postherpetic neuralgia*

# Malignant melanoma

- Neoplasm that arises from melanocytes, characterized by enlargement of skin lesion or nevus accompanied by changes in color, inflammation, soreness, itching, ulceration, bleeding, or textural changes
- Common sites: head and neck (men), legs (women), and back (those exposed to excessive sunlight); up to 70% arise from preexisting nevus
- Classified as superficial spreading melanoma, nodular malignant melanoma, lentigo maligna melanoma, and acral-lentiginous melanoma
- Increased incidence (up 50% in past 20 years) suggests earlier detection
- About 10 times more common among white populations

**THE PATHO PICTURE**

## HOW MALIGNANT MELANOMA DEVELOPS

A malignant neoplasm that arises from melanocytes, malignant melanoma can arise on normal skin or from an existing mole. If not treated promptly, it can spread through the lymphatic and vascular system and metastasize to the regional lymph nodes, skin, liver, lungs, and central nervous system. The illustrations below show a cross-section of a malignant melanoma and its defining characteristics.

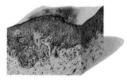

**Asymmetry**

**Borders**

**Diameter**

6 mm

## *Causes*

◆ Excessive exposure to ultraviolet light
◆ History of blistering sunburn before age 20
◆ Skin type:
   – in whites, typically blond or red hair, fair skin, blue eyes, prone to sunburn; Celtic or Scandinavian descent
   – in blacks, usually arises in lightly pigmented areas (palms, plantar surface of feet, or mucous membranes)
◆ Genetic or autoimmune factors
◆ Hormonal factors (pregnancy may increase risk and exacerbate growth)
◆ Family history
◆ History of melanoma (recurrence 10 times more likely)

## ▲ *Pathophysiologic changes*

### SUPERFICIAL SPREADING MELANOMA

Mutation in melanin-producing cells of skin ➡️

Develops on chronically sun-exposed areas, such as legs, upper back (usually within a nevus)
– Appears as red, white, or blue in color over a brown or black background, with irregular, notched margin
– Has irregular, small, elevated tumor nodules that may ulcerate and bleed
– Horizontal growth may continue for years; when vertical growth begins, prognosis worsens

### NODULAR MALIGNANT MELANOMA

Mutation in melanin-producing cells of skin ➡️

Resembles blood blister or polyp (most frequently misdiagnosed melanoma)
– More common in men
– May appear anywhere on body

*(continued)*

## *Pathophysiologic changes (continued)*

### LENTIGO MALIGNA MELANOMA

Mutation in melanin-producing
cells of skin ➡

Commonly develops under fingernails, on face, and on backs of hands
– Resembles large (1″ to 2″ [2.5 to 5 cm]), flat freckle of tan, brown, black, whitish, or slate color, with irregularly scattered black nodules on surface
– Develops slowly (over many years) and eventually may ulcerate

### ACRAL-LENTIGINOUS MELANOMA

Mutation in melanin-producing
cells of skin ➡

Develops as irregular, enlarging black macule
– Occurs mainly on palms and soles (especially on tip of finger or toe or in nail fold or bed)
– Most common among Asian and black populations

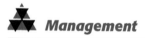 *Management*

- Surgical resection (extent of resection depends on size and location of primary tumor; may require skin graft) — *to remove tumor*
- Regional lymphadenectomy — *to help prevent metastasis*
- Chemotherapy or biotherapy (for deep primary lesions) — *to eliminate or reduce number of tumor cells*
- Radiation therapy or gene therapy — *for metastatic disease*
- Long-term follow-up — *to detect metastasis and recurrences*
- Patient teaching and recommendation of sun block use — *to help prevent recurrence*

# Psoriasis

◆ Chronic, recurrent disease characterized by epidermal proliferation, with recurring partial remissions and exacerbations
◆ Flare-ups commonly related to specific systemic and environmental factors, but may be unpredictable
◆ Exfoliative or erythrodermic psoriasis signifies widespread involvement

**THE PATHO PICTURE**

## UNDERSTANDING PSORIASIS

Psoriasis is a chronic, noncontagious inflammatory skin disease marked by reddish papules (solid elevations) and plaques covered with silvery scales. Psoriatic skin cells have a shortened maturation time as they migrate from the basal membrane to the surface or stratum corneum. As a result, the stratum corneum develops thick, scaly plaques, the chief sign of psoriasis.

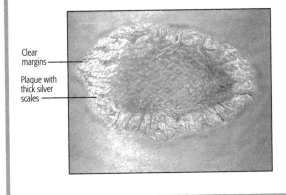

Clear margins ——

Plaque with thick silver scales ——

## *Causes*

- ◆ Genetic factors
- ◆ Possible immune disorder (associated with presence of human leukocyte antigens)
- ◆ Environmental factors
- ◆ Isomorphic effect or Koebner's phenomenon (lesions develop at sites of injury due to trauma)
- ◆ Beta-hemolytic streptococcal infections (associated with certain flare-ups)
- ◆ Pregnancy
- ◆ Endocrine changes
- ◆ Climate (cold weather tends to exacerbate psoriasis)
- ◆ Emotional stress

## ▲ *Pathophysiologic changes*

| | |
|---|---|
| Immune-based inflammatory reaction by T-cells in dermis ➡ | Erythematous and usually well-defined plaques, sometimes covering large areas of body (psoriatic lesions)<br>– Lesions most commonly appear on scalp, chest, elbows, knees, back, and buttocks<br>– Plaques have characteristic silver scales that either flake off easily or thicken, covering lesion; scale removal can produce fine bleeding<br>– Occasional small guttate lesions (usually thin and erythematous, with few scales), either alone or with plaques, appear |
| Dry, encrusted lesions ➡ | Itching and occasional pain (most common symptom) |

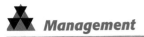

## Management

◆ Ultraviolet B (UVB) or natural sunlight exposure — *to retard rapid cell production to point of minimal erythema*

◆ Topical therapy (steroid creams and ointments, anthralin ointment, calcipotriene ointment, coal tar, tazarotene) — *to control symptoms of psoriasis*

◆ Goeckerman regimen (combines tar baths and UVB treatments) — *to help achieve remission and clear skin in 3 to 5 weeks (severe chronic psoriasis)*

◆ Psoralens (plant extracts that accelerate exfoliation) with exposure to high-intensity ultraviolet A (UVA) (psoralen plus UVA [PUVA] therapy) — *to retard rapid cell production*

◆ Immunomodulators (Alefacept, methotrexate, cyclosporine) — *to treat extensive, widespread, or resistant disease*

◆ Retinoids (Acitretin, tazarotene) — *to stimulate cell differentiation and inhibit malignant transformation in skin*

◆ Low-dose antihistamines, oatmeal baths, emollients, and open wet dressings — *to help relieve pruritus*

◆ Referral to National Psoriasis Foundation — *for information and support*

# Squamous cell carcinoma

♦ Invasive tumor with metastatic potential that arises from keratinizing epidermal cells
♦ Occurs most often in fair-skinned white men over age 60
♦ Higher incidence with outdoor employment or residence in sunny, warm climate

**THE PATHO PICTURE**

### HOW SQUAMOUS CELL CARCINOMA DEVELOPS

Squamous cell carcinoma is an invasive tumor with metastatic potential that arises from the keratinizing epidermal cells. It begins as a firm, red nodule or scaly, crusted flat lesion that may remain confined to the epidermis for a period of time. It eventually spreads to the dermis; untreated, it will spread to regional lymph nodes.

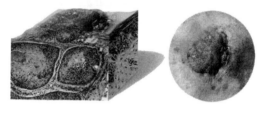

## Causes

♦ Common predisposing factors:
   – overexposure to sun's ultraviolet rays
   – presence of premalignant lesions (actinic keratosis or Bowen's disease)
♦ Other factors:
   – X-ray therapy
   – ingestion of herbicides containing arsenic
   – chronic skin irritation and inflammation, burns, or scars
   – exposure to local carcinogens (tar, oil)
   – hereditary diseases (xeroderma pigmentosum, albinism)
♦ Site of smallpox vaccination, psoriasis, or chronic discoid lupus erythematosus (rare)

# ▲ *Pathophysiologic changes*

| | |
|---|---|
| Mutation in keratinizing epidermal cells of skin ➡ | Nodule with firm, indurated base |
| Inflammation and induration of lesion ➡ | Early lesions: Scaling and ulceration of opaque, firm nodules with indistinct borders; may appear on face, ear, dorsa of hand and forearm, or other sun-damaged area |
| Keratinization ➡ | Later lesions: Scaly; most common on face and hands (sun-exposed areas); lesion on lower lip or ear may indicate invasive metastasis (generally poor prognosis) |
| Metastasis to regional lymph nodes ➡ | Pain, malaise, fatigue, weakness, and anorexia |

# ▲ *Management*

- ◆ Surgical excision — *to remove lesion*
- ◆ Electrodesiccation and curettage (which offer good cosmetic results for small lesions) — *to remove lesion*
- ◆ Radiation therapy (generally for elderly or debilitated patients) — *to remove lesion*
- ◆ Chemosurgery (reserved for resistant or recurrent lesions) — *to remove lesion*
- ◆ Instructions on avoiding excessive sun exposure, wearing protective clothing, and use of sunscreen (containing para-aminobenzoic acid, benzophenone, and zinc) and lip balm — *to minimize risk of future sun damage*

# 11

# Reproductive disorders

## Pathophysiologic concepts   269

## Disorders   271

# PATHOPHYSIOLOGIC CONCEPTS

## *Hormonal alterations*

◆ Defect or malfunction of hypothalamic-pituitary-ovarian axis system (in females)
  – May cause infertility due to insufficient gonadotropin secretions (both LH and FSH)
  – Possible causes of insufficient gonadotropin levels: infections, tumors, neurologic disease of hypothalamus or pituitary gland
  – Ovarian control related to system of negative and positive feedback mediated by estrogen production
  – Sporadic inhibition of ovulation related to hormonal imbalance in gonadotropin production and regulation, or abnormalities in adrenal or thyroid gland that adversely affect hypothalamic-pituitary functioning
◆ Male hypogonadism (abnormal decrease in gonad size and function) results from decreased androgen production
  – May impair spermatogenesis, causing infertility
  – May inhibit development of normal secondary sex characteristics

## *Male structural alterations*

◆ Structural defects may be congenital or acquired
◆ Benign prostatic hyperplasia (common with aging) involves prostate enlargement due to androgen-induced growth of prostate cells; may result in urinary obstructive symptoms
◆ Urethral stricture involves narrowing of urethra from scarring related to trauma, surgery (adhesions), or infection

## *Menstrual alterations*

◆ Menopause marks cessation of ovarian function
  – Results from complex continuum of physiologic changes (climacteric) caused by normal, gradual decline of ovarian function
  – Most dramatic climacteric change: cessation of menses
◆ Premature menopause (gradual or abrupt cessation of menses before age 35) occurs without apparent cause; affects about 5% of women in United States
◆ Artificial menopause may follow radiation therapy or surgical procedures, such as removal of both ovaries (bilateral oophorectomy)
◆ Ovarian failure (no ova produced) may result from functional ovarian disorder caused by premature menopause; amenorrhea ensues

# DISORDERS

## Benign prostatic hyperplasia

◆ Characterized by enlargement of prostate gland and compression of urethra, causing overt urinary obstruction; also known as benign prostatic hypertrophy

◆ Typically associated with aging (most men over age 50 have some prostatic enlargement)

◆ Treated symptomatically or surgically, depending on prostate size, age and health of patient, and extent of obstruction

**THE PATHO PICTURE**

### UNDERSTANDING BENIGN PROSTATIC HYPERPLASIA

Regardless of the cause, benign prostatic hyperplasia begins with nonmalignant changes in periurethral glandular tissue. The growth of the fibroadenomatous nodules (masses of fibrous glandular tissue) progresses to compress the remaining normal gland (nodular hyperplasia). The hyperplastic tissue is mostly glandular, with some fibrous stroma and smooth muscle. As the prostate enlarges, it may extend into the bladder and obstruct urinary outflow by compressing or distorting the prostatic urethra. Progressive bladder distention may also cause a pouch to form in the bladder that retains urine when the rest of the bladder empties. This retained urine may lead to calculus formation or cystitis.

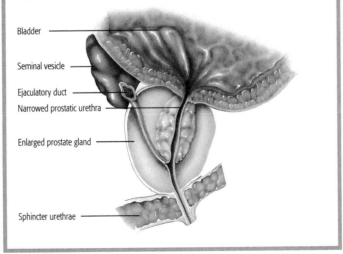

Bladder

Seminal vesicle

Ejaculatory duct

Narrowed prostatic urethra

Enlarged prostate gland

Sphincter urethrae

## *Causes*

◆ Exact cause unknown
◆ Possible age-related changes in hormone activity: androgenic hormone production decreases with age, causing imbalance in androgen and estrogen levels and high levels of dihydrotestosterone (main prostatic intracellular androgen)

## *Risk factors*

◆ Aging
◆ Family history

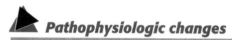 *Pathophysiologic changes*

| | |
|---|---|
| Enlarged prostate ➡ | Reduced urinary stream caliber and force; urinary hesitancy; difficulty starting micturition (straining, feeling of incomplete voiding, and interrupted stream) |
| Increased obstruction and prostate size ➡ | Frequent urination with nocturia; dribbling; urine retention; incontinence; sense of urgency; possible hematuria |

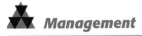

## *Management*

- Alpha-adrenergic blockers (terazosin [Hytrin], prazosin [Minipress])— *to improve urine flow and relieve bladder outlet obstruction by preventing contractions of prostatic capsule and bladder neck*
- Finasteride (Proscar) — *to possibly reduce prostate size*
- Antimicrobials — *to treat infection*
- Continuous drainage with indwelling urinary catheter — *to alleviate urine retention (when other treatment measures ineffective)*
- Transurethral, suprapubic (transvesical), or retropubic (extravesical) resection — *to remove prostate gland*
- Balloon dilation of urethra and prostatic stents — *to maintain urethral patency (occasionally)*
- Laser excision — *to relieve prostatic enlargement*
- Nerve-sparing surgical techniques — *to reduce common complications (erectile dysfunction)*
- Prostate massages, sitz baths, fluid restriction — *to prevent bladder distention*
- Regular ejaculation — *to help relieve prostatic congestion*
- Saw palmetto (herbal remedy) — *to help improve urine flow and relieve nocturia*

# Breast cancer

♦ Most common cancer affecting women
♦ May develop anytime after puberty; most common after age 50

**THE PATHO PICTURE**

▼**CELLULAR PROGRESSION OF BREAST CANCER**

Breast cancer is more common in the left breast than in the right and more common in the upper outer quadrant. Growth rates vary. It spreads by way of the lymphatic system and bloodstream to the other breast, the chest wall, liver, bone, and brain.

Classified by histologic appearance and the lesion's location, breast cancer may be described as follows:

♦ *adenocarcinoma* – arising from the epithelium
♦ *intraductal* – developing within the ducts (includes Paget's disease)
♦ *infiltrating* – occurring in parenchymal tissue
♦ *inflammatory* (rare) – rapidly growing and causing overlying skin to become edematous, inflamed, and indurated
♦ *lobular carcinoma in situ* – involving lobes of glandular tissue
♦ *medullary or circumscribed* – enlarging rapidly.

Breast cancer originates in the epithelial lining of the breast. This illustration shows the intraductal changes, with transformation of benign cells to atypical cells to malignant cells.

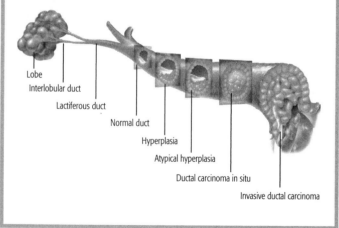

Lobe
Interlobular duct
Lactiferous duct
Normal duct
Hyperplasia
Atypical hyperplasia
Ductal carcinoma in situ
Invasive ductal carcinoma

## Causes

◆ Unknown, but its high incidence in women implicates estrogen
◆ Possible causes: estrogen therapy, antihypertensive agents, high-fat diet, obesity, fibrocystic breast disease

## Risk factors

◆ Factors associated with high risk:
  – family history of breast cancer, particularly first-degree relative (mother or sister)
  – genetic mutations in BRCA-1 and BRCA-2 genes (suggest genetic predisposition)
  – long menses (began menses early or menopause late)
  – no history of pregnancy
  – first pregnancy after age 30
  – history of unilateral breast cancer
  – history of endometrial or ovarian cancer
  – exposure to low-level ionizing radiation
◆ Factors associated with lower risk:
  – history of pregnancy before age 20
  – history of multiple pregnancies
  – Native American or Asian ethnicity

# ▲ *Pathophysiologic changes*

| | |
|---|---|
| Mutation in cells of breast tissue ▶ | Lump or mass in breast (hard, stony mass is usually malignant); change in breast size or symmetry; change in nipple (itching, burning, erosion, or retraction) and nipple discharge (watery, serous, creamy, bloody) |
| Fixation of cancer to pectoral muscles or underlying fascia ▶ | Change in breast skin (thickening, scaly skin around nipple, dimpling) |
| Edema ▶ | Change in skin texture (peau d'orange) |
| Advanced spread within breast ▶ | Change in skin temperature (warm, hot, or pink area), ulceration, edema, or pain (not usually present; should be investigated) |
| Metastasis ▶ | Pathologic bone fractures, edema of arm |

# 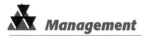 *Management*

### SURGICAL TREATMENT

◆ Lumpectomy (may be combined with radiation therapy); lumpectomy and dissection of axillary lymph nodes; simple mastectomy; modified radical mastectomy; radical mastectomy — *to remove diseased tissue*

◆ Reconstructive surgery (may follow mastectomy) — *to restore normal anatomical appearance and improve self-esteem*

### MEDICAL TREATMENT

◆ Chemotherapy (cyclophosphamide, fluorouracil, methotrexate, doxorubicin, vincristine, paclitaxel, prednisone) — *to kill cancer cells*

◆ Tamoxifen — *as adjuvant treatment of choice for postmenopausal patients with positive estrogen receptor status*

◆ Peripheral stem cell therapy — *to treat advanced breast cancer*

◆ Primary radiation therapy — *for small tumors in early stages with no evidence of distant metastasis; also used to prevent or treat local recurrence*

◆ Presurgical radiation (in patients with inflammatory breast cancer) — *to help make tumors more surgically manageable*

◆ Palliative treatment (pain management and radiation therapy) for bone metastasis — *to maintain patient comfort*

### OTHER MEASURES

◆ Referral to American Cancer Society's Reach to Recovery program — *to provide instruction, emotional support, counseling, and information about breast prostheses*

◆ Patient teaching about clinical breast examination and mammography (following American Cancer Society guidelines) — *to provide information about breast cancer detection*

# Endometriosis

◆ Presence of endometrial tissue outside lining of uterine cavity (ectopic tissue)
◆ Generally confined to pelvic area (usually around ovaries, uterovesical peritoneum, uterosacral ligaments, and cul de sac) but can appear anywhere in body (including intestines, even found in lungs and limbs)
◆ Classic symptoms: dysmenorrhea, abnormal uterine bleeding, and infertility

**THE PATHO PICTURE**

### UNDERSTANDING ENDOMETRIOSIS

Ectopic endometrial tissue can implant almost anywhere in the peritoneum. It responds to normal stimulation in the same way as the endometrium, but more unpredictably. The endometrial cells respond to estrogen and progesterone with proliferation and secretion. During menstruation, the ectopic tissue bleeds, which causes inflammation of the surrounding tissues. This inflammation causes fibrosis, leading to adhesions that produce pain and infertility.

This illustration shows endometrial implants and a ruptured endometrial cyst.

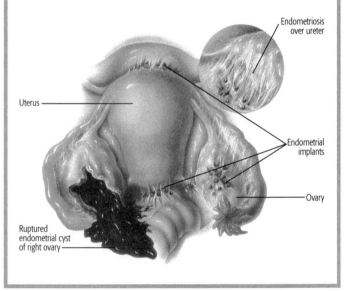

Endometriosis over ureter

Uterus

Endometrial implants

Ovary

Ruptured endometrial cyst of right ovary

## *Causes*

◆ Exact cause unknown
◆ May be related to:
– retrograde menstruation with endometrial implantation at ectopic sites
– genetic predisposition and depressed immune system
– coelomic metaplasia (repeated inflammation inducing metaplasia of mesothelial cells to endometrial epithelium)
– lymphatic or hematogenous spread (extraperitoneal disease)

## ▲ *Pathophysiologic changes*

| | |
|---|---|
| Implantation of ectopic tissue and adhesions ▶ | **Dysmenorrhea**<br>– Pain typically begins 5 to 7 days before menses, lasts for 2 to 3 days after peak of menses<br>– Intensity varies depending on location of ectopic tissue |
| Ectopic tissue in ovaries and oviducts ▶ | **Infertility and profuse menses** |
| Ectopic tissue in ovaries or cul de sac ▶ | **Deep-thrust dyspareunia** |
| Ectopic tissue in bladder ▶ | **Suprapubic pain, dysuria, and hematuria** |
| Ectopic tissue in large bowel and appendix ▶ | **Abdominal cramps, pain on defecation, constipation; bloody stools (from bleeding of ectopic endometrium in rectosigmoid musculature)** |
| Ectopic tissue in cervix, vagina, and peritoneum ▶ | **Bleeding from endometrial deposits during menses; painful intercourse** |

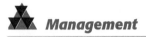 *Management*

◆ Androgens (danazol [Danocrine]) — *to slow growth of endometrial tissue outside uterus*
◆ Progestins and continuous combined hormonal contraceptives (pseudopregnancy regimen) — *to relieve symptoms by causing regression of endometrial tissue*
◆ GnRH agonists — *to induce pseudomenopause (medical oophorectomy), causing remission*
◆ Mild analgesics or nonsteroidal anti-inflammatory agents — *for pain management*
◆ Laparoscopic surgery (with conventional or laser techniques) — *to remove endometrial implants*
◆ Presacral neurectomy — *for central pelvic pain*
◆ Laparoscopic uterosacral nerve ablation (LUNA) — *for central pelvic pain*
◆ Total abdominal hysterectomy (with or without bilateral salpingo-oophorectomy) — *as treatment of last resort for women who don't want to have children or for extensive disease*

# Herpes simplex type 2

◆ Recurrent viral infection caused by *Herpesvirus hominis*
◆ Also known as genital herpes
   – Primarily affects genital area; commonly transmitted by sexual contact
   – Cross-infection may result from orogenital sex
◆ Characterized by painful, fluid-filled vesicles that appear in genital area (some cases remain subclinical, with no symptoms)
◆ Treatment is largely supportive; no known cure

---

### HOW IT HAPPENS

Commonly known as genital herpes, herpes simplex type 2 is transmitted by contact with infectious lesions or secretions. The virus enters the skin, local replication of the virus occurs, and the virus enters cutaneous neurons. After the patient becomes infected, a latency period follows, although repeated outbreaks may develop at any time.

**Initial Infection**
Highly infectious period, with manifestation of symptoms after incubation period (average period: 1 week)

**Latency**
Intermittently infectious period, marked by viral dormancy or viral shedding and no disease symptoms

**Recurrent infection**
Highly infectious period similar to initial infection, with milder symptoms that resolve faster

## *Causes*

- ◆ Transmission of *Herpesvirus hominis* (causes both type 1 and type 2 herpes)
  - – primarily by sexual contact
  - – possibly by autoinocculation with type 1 herpes (through poor hand-washing practices or orogenital sex)
- ◆ Pregnancy-related transmission (infected pregnant patient may transmit virus to newborn during vaginal delivery; cesarean section recommended during initial infection when active lesions are present)

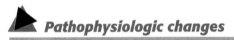

## *Pathophysiologic changes*

| | |
|---|---|
| Viral penetration of skin, viral replication, and entry into cutaneous neurons ➡ | Initial symptoms: pain, tingling and itching in genital area, followed by eruption of localized, fluid-filled vesicles |
| Painful lesions ➡ | Dysuria and dyspareunia |
| Progression of viral infection ➡ | Malaise, fever, leukorrhea (in females), and lymphadenopathy |

## *Management*

- ◆ Antiviral drugs (acyclovir, valacyclovir, famciclovir) — *to decrease severity and shorten duration of lesions, decrease viral shedding, and decrease frequency of recurrence*
- ◆ Analgesics and antipyretics — *to reduce fever and relieve pain*
- ◆ Warm baths, cool compresses, or topical anesthetics — *to help reduce pain*
- ◆ Education and counseling — *to provide patient with information about care measures during outbreaks, prevention of secondary or recurrent herpes infections (including eye infections), measures to avoid infecting others (avoiding sexual activity during active stage, using condoms), and risks of fetal infection*

# Prostate cancer

- ◆ Slow-growing, most common neoplasm in men over age 50
- ◆ Commonly forms as adenocarcinoma (derived from glandular tissue); sarcomas rarely occur
- ◆ Usually originates in posterior prostate gland; sometimes originates near urethra
- ◆ Seldom results from benign hyperplastic enlargement (common with aging)
- ◆ Clinical manifestations typically associated with later stages of disease

**THE PATHO PICTURE**

### HOW PROSTATE CANCER DEVELOPS

Prostate cancer (commonly a form of adenocarcinoma) grows slowly. When primary lesions metastasize beyond the prostate, they invade the prostate capsule and spread along the ejaculatory ducts in the space between the seminal vesicles.

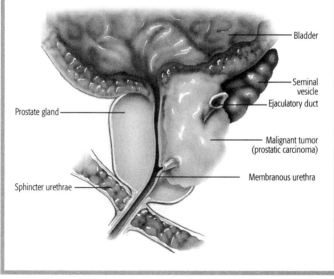

## *Causes*

♦ Exact cause unknown
♦ Predisposing factors:
  – aging (incidence rapidly increases after age 50)
  – genetic component (risk increases in men having first-degree relative with prostate cancer)
  – ethnic origin (highest reported incidence in African American men)
  – exposure to environmental and occupational toxins

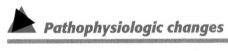

### *Pathophysiologic changes*

| | |
|---|---|
| Obstruction of urinary tract by tumor ➡ | **Difficulty initiating urinary stream, dribbling, urine retention, unexplained cystitis** |
| Infiltration of bladder by tumor ➡ | **Hematuria** |
| Bone metastasis ➡ | **Back pain** |

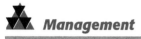

# Management

- ◆ Radiation therapy — *to treat locally invasive lesions (may also relieve bone pain associated with metastasis)*
- ◆ Radioactive seed implants into prostate (brachytherapy) — *to enhance radiation of cancerous area with minimal exposure to surrounding tissue*
- ◆ Hormonal therapy (flutamide) — *to treat androgen-dependent prostate cancer*
- ◆ Radical prostatectomy — *to remove prostate gland and tumor*
- ◆ Transurethral resection of prostate — *to relieve obstruction*
- ◆ Orchiectomy — *to decrease androgen production*
- ◆ Cryoablation — *to remove tumor by freezing*
- ◆ Pain management — *to alleviate pain associated with bone metastasis*

# Toxic shock syndrome

- ◆ Acute bacterial infection caused by toxin-producing, penicillin-resistant strains of *Staphylococcus aureus* (TSS toxin-1 and staphylococcal enterotoxins B and C)
- ◆ Primarily affects menstruating women under age 30
- ◆ Associated with continuous use of tampons during menstrual period
- ◆ Incidence peaked in mid-1980s; has since declined (probably because of withdrawal of high-absorbency tampons)

---

### HOW IT HAPPENS

Toxic shock syndrome is an acute bacterial infection caused by toxin-producing, penicillin-resistant strains of *Staphylococcus aureus*. It is primarily associated with continuous use of tampons during the menstrual period, although some cases unrelated to tampon use have been reported. Toxin-producing bacterial pathogens are introduced into the vagina by way of contaminated fingers or tampon applicator, and the menstrual flow provides a medium for bacterial growth.

| Toxin-producing bacteria enter host. |
| --- |

| Exotoxins are released from bacterial cell during growth; their enzymatic activity damage host cell. |
| --- |

| Bacteria multiply, producing large quantities of exotoxins. |
| --- |

| Exotoxins diffuse from the hyperemic vaginal mucosa and enter the bloodstream; as compensatory mechanisms fail, the shock state occurs. |
| --- |

## *Causes*

◆ Tampon-related mechanism:
  – introduction of *S. aureus* into vagina during insertion
  – vaginal absorption of toxin after insertion
  – traumatization of vaginal mucosa during insertion
  – favorable environment conducive to growth of *S. aureus*
◆ Infection of *S. aureus* unrelated to menstruation:
  – abscess
  – osteomyelitis
  – postsurgical infections
  – use of contraceptive devices (diaphragms, sponges)
  – recent childbirth

## ▲ *Pathophysiologic changes*

| | |
|---|---|
| Toxin-producing infection ➡ | Intense myalgias, fever over 104° F (40° C), vomiting, diarrhea, headache, decreased level of consciousness, vaginal hyperemia and discharge |
| Hypersensitivity reaction to toxin ➡ | Deep-red rash (especially on palms and soles)<br>– Develops within hours of onset<br>– Desquamates later |
| Disease progression ➡ | Severe hypotension, hypovolemic shock, possible renal failure |

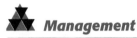

## Management

- Beta-lactamase-resistant antistaphylococcal antibiotics (oxacillin, nafcillin) given I.V. — *to eliminate infection*
- Fluid replacement with I.V. solution and colloids — *to reverse shock*
- Pressor agents (dopamine) — *to treat shock unresponsive to fluid replacement*
- Dialysis (may be necessary) — *for kidney dysfunction*
- I.V. immunoglobulin (in some cases) — *to neutralize circulating toxins*

# 12

# Genetic disorders

# PATHOPHYSIOLOGIC CONCEPTS

## *Chromosome defects*

◆ Responsible for congenital anomalies (birth defects)
◆ May involve loss, addition, or rearrangement of genetic material
◆ Development of clinically significant aberrations linked with meiosis
◆ Translocation (shifting or moving of chromosomal material) occurs when chromosomes split apart and rejoin in abnormal arrangement

## *Gene errors*

◆ Permanent change in genetic material (mutation)
◆ May occur anywhere in genome (entire inventory of genes)
◆ May occur spontaneously or after cellular exposure to radiation, certain chemicals, or viruses
◆ If not identified or repaired, may produce trait different from original and transmit to offspring during reproduction

### AUTOSOMAL DISORDERS

◆ Results from error that occurs at single gene site on deoxyribonucleic acid (DNA) strand
◆ Inherited in clearly identifiable patterns (same as with inheritance of normal traits)
  – chance of inheritance depends on whether one or both parents have affected gene
  – usually, males and females have equal chance of inheriting disorder
◆ Involves transmission of either dominant gene (autosomal dominant inheritance) or recessive gene (autosomal recessive inheritance); autosomal recessive disorders may occur with no family history of disease

### MULTIFACTORIAL DISORDERS

◆ Commonly result from effects of several different genes and an environmental component
◆ Sometimes apparent at birth (cleft lip, cleft palate, congenital heart disease, anencephaly, clubfoot, myelomeningocele); may manifest later (type II diabetes, hypertension, hyperlipidemia, autoimmune disease, cancer)

### SEX-LINKED DISORDERS

◆ Caused by genetic error located on sex chromosomes (most commonly X chromosome, usually involving transmission of recessive trait)
◆ Patterns of transmission differ with males and females
  – males (only one X chromosome): single X-linked recessive gene can cause disease
  – females (two X chromosomes): can be homozygous for disease allele, homozygous for normal allele, or heterozygous (carrier)
◆ Person with abnormal trait typically has one affected parent; most common transmission is from union of carrier female and normal male
◆ Involves inheritance of dominant or recessive gene (most dominant disorders are lethal in males)
  – when father is affected (either dominant or recessive gene): all daughters will be affected (dominant gene) or carriers (recessive gene); all sons will be unaffected or noncarriers
  – when mother is carrier (recessive gene): unaffected sons will not transmit disorder
  – when mother is affected (dominant gene): each child has 50% chance of being affected

# DISORDERS

## Cystic fibrosis

◆ Chronic, progressive dysfunction of exocrine glands that affects multiple organ systems
◆ Most common fatal genetic disease in white children (typically of northern European descent)
◆ Carries average life expectancy of 32 years
◆ Characterized by chronic airway infection leading to bronchiectasis, bronchiolectasis, exocrine pancreatic insufficiency, intestinal dysfunction, abnormal sweat gland function, and reproductive dysfunction

### HOW IT HAPPENS

Cystic fibrosis typically arises from a mutation in the genetic coding of a single amino acid found in a protein called cystic fibrosis transmembrane regulator (CFTR). This protein, which is involved in the transport of chloride and other ions across cell membranes, resembles other transmembrane transport proteins but lacks phenylalanine (an essential amino acid in protein produced by normal genes) and therefore doesn't function properly.

Mutation in coding of amino acid

Interference with cAMP-regulated chloride channels and transport of other ions by preventing adenosine triphosphate (ATP) from binding to the CFTR protein or by interfering with activation by protein kinase

Epithelial dysfunction in airways and intestines (volume-absorbing epithelia), sweat ducts (salt-absorbing epithelia), and pancreas (volume-secretory epithelia)

Dehydration, increased viscosity of mucus secretions, and obstruction of glandular ducts

## *Cause*

◆ Genetic mutation on chromosome 7q
  – may involve as many as 350 alleles within cystic fibrosis transmembrane regulator protein (CFTR)
  – transmitted by autosomal recessive inheritance

## ▲ *Pathophysiologic changes*

| | |
|---|---|
| Ionic imbalance ▶ | **Thick secretions and dehydration** |
| Abnormal airway surface fluids and failure of lung defenses ▶ | **Chronic airway infections (***Staphylococcus aureus, Pseudomonas aeruginosa,* **and** *P. cepacia***)** |
| Accumulation of thick secretions in bronchioles and alveoli ▶ | **Dyspnea, paroxysmal cough, crackles, wheezes** |
| Chronic hypoxia ▶ | **Barrel chest, cyanosis, clubbing of fingers and toes** |
| Absence of CFTR chloride channel in pancreatic ductile epithelia ▶ | **Retention of bicarbonate and water (leads to retention of pancreatic enzymes, chronic cholecystitis and cholelithiasis, and ultimate destruction of pancreas)** |
| Inhibited secretion of chloride and water and excessive absorption of liquid ▶ | **Obstruction of small and large intestine** |
| Retention of biliary secretions ▶ | **Biliary cirrhosis** |
| Hyponatremia and hypochloremia from sodium lost in sweat ▶ | **Fatal shock and arrhythmias** |
| Malabsorption of nutrients ▶ | **Failure to thrive: poor weight gain, poor growth, distended abdomen, thin extremities, and sallow skin with poor turgor** |
| Deficiency of fat-soluble vitamins ▶ | **Clotting problems, retarded bone growth, delayed sexual development** |

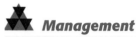

## Management

- ◆ Hypertonic radiocontrast materials delivered by enema — *to treat acute obstructions due to meconium ileus*
- ◆ Breathing exercises, postural drainage, and chest percussion — *to clear pulmonary secretions*
- ◆ Antibiotics — *to treat lung infection (guided by sputum culture results)*
- ◆ Bronchodilators and mucolytic agents — *to control airway constriction and to increase mucus clearance*
- ◆ Pancreatic enzyme replacement — *to maintain adequate nutrition*
- ◆ Sodium-channel blockers — *to decrease sodium resorption from secretions and improve viscosity*
- ◆ Uridine triphosphate — *to stimulate chloride secretion by non-CFTR proteins*
- ◆ Sodium supplements — *to replace electrolytes lost through sweat*
- ◆ Dornase alfa (genetically engineered pulmonary enzyme) — *to help liquefy mucus*
- ◆ Recombinant alpha-antitrypsin — *to counteract excessive proteolytic activity produced during airway inflammation*
- ◆ Gene therapy — *to introduce normal CFTR into affected epithelial cells*
- ◆ Transplantation of heart or lungs — *for severe organ failure*
- ◆ Referral for genetic counseling (Cystic Fibrosis Foundation) — *to discuss family planning issues or prenatal diagnosis options*

# Down syndrome

◆ Spontaneous chromosome abnormality that causes characteristic facial features and other distinctive physical abnormalities (apparent at birth) and mental retardation

◆ Also called trisomy 21 (chromosome defect appears on chromosome 21)

◆ Carries significantly increased life expectancy due to improved treatment for heart defects, respiratory and other infections, and acute leukemia

**THE PATHO PICTURE**

### UNDERSTANDING DOWN SYNDROME

Human chromosomes are arranged in seven groups, designated by the letters A through G. The illustrations below and on the next page show the arrangement of chromosomes (karyotype) in a normal person and a person with Down syndrome (trisomy 21). In most cases of Down syndrome, there's an extra chromosome (chromosome 21 has three copies instead of two).

**Normal male**

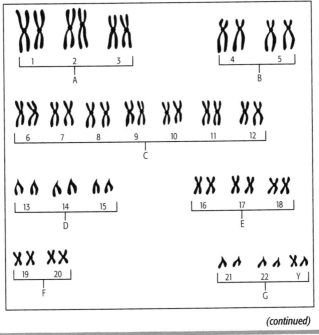

*(continued)*

**UNDERSTANDING DOWN SYNDROME** *(continued)*

**Male with Down syndrome**

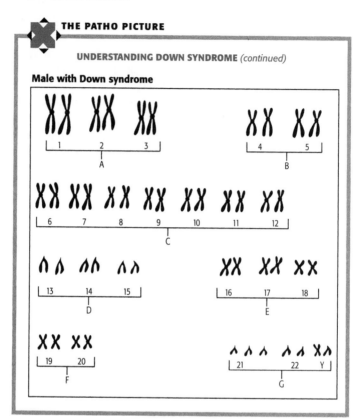

## Cause

◆ Chromosomal aberration (three copies of chromosome 21)

## Risk factors

◆ Advanced parental age (mother age 35 or older at delivery; father age 42 or older)
◆ Cumulative effects of environmental factors (radiation, viruses)

# ▲ *Pathophysiologic changes*

### CHARACTERISTIC PHYSICAL FINDINGS

Chromosomal aberration ➤      Distinctive craniofacial features (apparent at birth)
– Low nasal bridge
– Epicanthal folds, protruding tongue, and low-set ears
– Small open mouth and disproportionately large tongue
– Single transverse crease on palm (simian crease)
– Small white spots on iris (Brushfield's spots)

Lethargy (apparent at birth)

Mental retardation (estimated IQ of 30 to 70)

Congenital defects (heart defects, duodenal atresia, Hirschsprung's disease, polydactyly, syndactyly)

### OTHER FINDINGS

Hypotonia and decreased cognitive processing ➤      Developmental delay

Decreased muscle tone in limbs ➤      Impaired reflexes

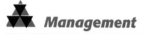 *Management*

♦ Surgery — *to correct heart defects and other related congenital abnormalities*
♦ Antibiotics — *for recurrent infections*
♦ Early intervention programs and supportive therapies — *to maximize mental and physical capabilities*
♦ Thyroid hormone replacement — *for hypothyroidism*
♦ Genetic and psychological counseling — *to evaluate future reproductive risks*
♦ Referral to national or local Down syndrome organizations and support groups — *for additional information and support*

# Hemophilia

♦ X-linked-inherited recessive bleeding disorder that results from deficiency of clotting factors
♦ Severity and prognosis of bleeding vary with degree of deficiency or nonfunction and site of bleeding
♦ Classification depends on clotting factor involved
  – Hemophilia A (classic hemophilia): deficiency of clotting factor VIII; affects more than 80% of those with hemophilia
  – Hemophilia B (Christmas disease): results from deficiency of factor IX; affects about 15% of those with disorder
♦ Prevention of crippling deformities and prolonged life expectancy possible with proper treatment

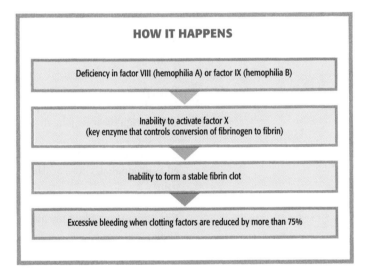

## HOW IT HAPPENS

Deficiency in factor VIII (hemophilia A) or factor IX (hemophilia B)

Inability to activate factor X
(key enzyme that controls conversion of fibrinogen to fibrin)

Inability to form a stable fibrin clot

Excessive bleeding when clotting factors are reduced by more than 75%

## *Cause*

♦ Chromosomal defect
  – specific gene on X chromosome that codes for factor VIII synthesis (hemophilia A)
  – substitution of more than 300 different base-pair genes on X chromosome that code for factor IX (hemophilia B)

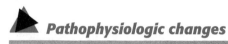

## Pathophysiologic changes

Lack of clotting factor ➡

Spontaneous bleeding (severe hemophilia)

Excessive or continued bleeding or bruising (after minor trauma or surgery)

Large subcutaneous and deep intramuscular hematomas (with mild trauma)

Prolonged bleeding (mild hemophilia after major trauma or surgery)

Pain, swelling, and tenderness (from bleeding into joints, especially weight-bearing joints)

Internal bleeding (often manifested as abdominal, chest, or flank pain)

Hematuria (from bleeding into kidney)

Hematemesis or tarry stools (from bleeding into GI tract)

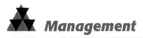 *Management*

♦ Cryoprecipitate (for hemophilia A) or lyophilized factor VIII or IX — *to increase clotting factor levels and permit normal hemostasis levels*

♦ Factor IX concentrate — for bleeding episodes in hemophilia B

♦ Aminocaproic acid (Amicar) — *to inhibit plasminogen activator substances during oral bleeding episodes*

♦ Prophylactic desmopressin (DDAVP) before dental procedures or minor surgery — *to release stored von Willebrand's factor and factor VIII, thereby reducing bleeding*

♦ Use of clothing with padded patches on knees and elbows (young children) — *to prevent injury that could lead to bleeding*

♦ Avoidance of contact sports (older children) — *to prevent injury that could lead to bleeding*

♦ Referral of patients and carriers for genetic counseling — *to discuss family planning issues*

# Marfan syndrome

◆ Rare degenerative disease of connective tissue resulting from elastin and collagen defects
◆ Causes ocular, skeletal, and cardiovascular anomalies
◆ Death attributed to cardiovascular complications (from early infancy to adulthood)

---

### HOW IT HAPPENS

Marfan syndrome is inherited as an autosomal dominant trait that has been mapped to a specific gene located on chromosome 15. This gene codes for fibrillin (small, abundant fibers found in large blood vessels and the suspensory ligaments of ocular lenses). Over 20 mutations have been identified.

Mutation in single allele of gene located on chromosome 15 (codes for fibrillin, a glycoprotein component of connective tissue)

Primarily causes skeletal malformations, ocular defects, and cardiac abnormalities; miscellaneous effects include thin body build (with little subcutaneous fat), striae over shoulders and buttocks, spontaneous pneumothorax, inguinal and incisional hernias, dilation of dural sac

| Skeletal malformations: | Ocular defects: | Cardiac abnormalities (most serious consequence): |
|---|---|---|
| Abnormal growth (increased height, long extremities) Arachnodactyly (spiderlike hands and fingers) Chest depression, protrusion, and asymmetry Scoliosis and kyphosis Arched palate Joint hypermobility | Lens displacement Elongated ocular globe Retinal detachments and tears | Valvular abnormalities Mitral valve prolapse Aortic regurgitation, dissection, or rupture |

## Causes
- Autosomal dominant mutation on chromosome 15
- Advanced paternal age (possible in about 15% of patients with no family history of disease)

### ▲ Pathophysiologic changes

| | |
|---|---|
| Excessive bone growth ▶ | Increased height, long extremities, arachnodactyly (long spider-like fingers); defects of sternum (funnel chest or pigeon breast), chest asymmetry, scoliosis, and kyphosis |
| Elongated ocular globe ▶ | Nearsightedness |
| Altered connective tissue ▶ | Valvular abnormalities (redundancy of leaflets, stretching of chordae tendineae, and dilation of valvulae annulus); mitral valve prolapse; joint hypermobility; lens displacement (ocular hallmark of syndrome) |
| Dilation of aortic root and ascending aorta ▶ | Aortic insufficiency |
| Weakening of medial layer of aorta ▶ | Aortic dissection |

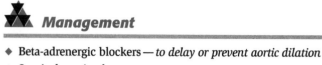

## Management

◆ Beta-adrenergic blockers — *to delay or prevent aortic dilation*
◆ Surgical repair of aneurysms — *to prevent rupture*
◆ Surgical correction of ocular deformities — *to improve vision*
◆ Steroid and sex hormone therapy — *to induce early epiphyseal closure and limit adult height*
◆ Surgical replacement of aortic valve and mitral valve — *for extreme dilation*
◆ Mechanical bracing and physical therapy — *for mild scoliosis (if curvature is greater than 20 degrees)*
◆ Surgical correction for scoliosis — *if curvature is greater than 45 degrees*
◆ Referral to National Marfan Foundation — *for additional information and support*

# Neural tube defects

- ◆ Congenital malformations that produce defects of spine or skull
- ◆ Result from failure of neural tube closure (normally occurs 24 to 28 days after conception)
- ◆ Most common forms: spina bifida, anencephaly, and encephalocele
- ◆ Spina bifida occulta is most common and least severe spinal cord defect

**THE PATHO PICTURE**

## UNDERSTANDING SPINAL CORD DEFECTS

Spina bifida occulta is characterized by a depression or raised area and a tuft of hair over the defect. Spina bifida cystica can take one of two forms: myelomeningocele or meningocele. In myelomeningocele, an external sac contains meninges, cerebrospinal fluid (CSF), and a portion of the spinal cord or nerve roots. In meningocele, an external sac contains only meninges and CSF.

**Spina bifida occulta**    **Myelo-meningocele**    **Meningocele**

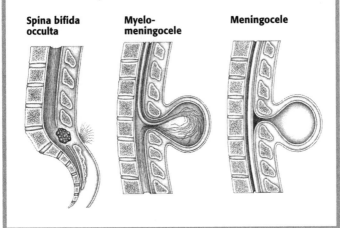

## *Causes*

◆ Exposure to teratogen
◆ Part of multiple malformation syndrome (chromosomal abnormalities, such as trisomy 18 or 13 syndrome)
◆ Combination of genetic and environmental factors (in isolated birth defects)
◆ Lack of dietary folic acid around time of conception

## *Pathophysiologic changes*

### SPINA BIFIDA OCCULTA

Incomplete closure of one or more vertebrae without protrusion of spinal cord or meninges ➡

Skin abnormalities over spinal defect (may appear alone or in combination): depression or dimple, tuft of hair, soft fatty deposits, port wine nevi

### SPINA BIFIDA CYSTICA

Incomplete closure of one or more vertebrae without protrusion of spinal contents ➡

Saclike structure protruding over spine, trophic skin disturbances, ulcerations

Spinal nerve roots ending at sac ➡

Neurologic dysfunction (depends on defect's location), possibly including spastic paralysis and bowel and bladder incontinence

### ENCEPHALOCELE

Saclike portion of meninges and brain protruding through defective opening in skull ➡

Paralysis, hydrocephalus, and mental retardation (findings vary with degree of tissue involvement and location of defect)

### ANENCEPHALY

Closure defect at cranial end of neuroaxis ➡

Exposed neural tissue, skull malformation (froglike appearance when viewed from front)

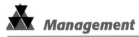 *Management*

◆ Surgical closure of protruding sac and continued assessment of growth and development (meningocele) — *to prevent further neurologic deficit*

◆ Sac repair and supportive measures — *to promote independence and prevent further complications (myelomeningocele)*

◆ Shunt — *to relieve associated hydrocephalus*

◆ Surgery during infancy — *to place protruding tissues back in skull, excise sac, and correct associated craniofacial abnormalities (encephalocele)*

◆ Rehabilitation measures (orthopedic appliances, bowel training, neurogenic bladder management) — *to promote independence and prevent further complications*

◆ Referral to Spina Bifida Association of America — *for genetic counseling and support*

# Sickle cell anemia

- ◆ Congenital hemolytic anemia resulting from defective hemoglobin molecules (hemoglobin S); produces characteristic sickle-shaped red blood cells (RBCs)
- ◆ Occurs primarily in those of African and Mediterranean descent
- ◆ Symptoms typically appear after age 6 months (due to presence of large amount of fetal hemoglobin)

**THE PATHO PICTURE**

## UNDERSTANDING SICKLE CELL CRISIS

Infection, exposure to cold, high altitudes, overexertion, or other situations that cause cellular oxygen deprivation may trigger a sickle cell crisis. The oxygenated, sickle-shaped red blood cells stick to the capillary wall and each other, blocking blood flow and causing cellular hypoxia. The crisis worsens as tissue hypoxia and acidic waste products cause more sickling and cell damage. With each new crisis, organs and tissues are slowly destroyed, especially the spleen and kidneys.

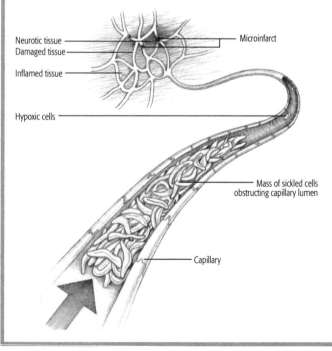

Neurotic tissue

Damaged tissue

Inflamed tissue

Hypoxic cells

Microinfarct

Mass of sickled cells obstructing capillary lumen

Capillary

## *Cause*

◆ Autosomal recessive inheritance (homozygous inheritance of hemoglobin S-producing gene)

 *Pathophysiologic changes*

| | |
|---|---|
| Repeated cycles of deoxygenation and sickling ➡ | **Anemia, tachycardia, cardiomegaly, chronic fatigue, unexplained dyspnea, hepatomegaly, joint swelling, aching bones** |
| Blood vessel obstruction by rigid, tangled, sickle cells (leading to tissue anoxia and possibly necrosis) ➡ | **Severe pain in abdomen, thorax, muscles, joints, or bones (characterizes painful crisis); pale lips, tongue, palms, or nail beds; lethargy; listlessness; sleepiness; irritability; severe pain; and fever** |
| Increased bilirubin production ➡ | **Jaundice, dark urine** |
| Autosplenectomy (splenic damage and scarring occurring with long-term disease) ➡ | **Susceptibility to infection, especially *Streptococcus pneumoniae*** |
| Bone marrow depression and infection (usually viral) ➡ | **Aplastic (megaloblastic) crisis: pallor, lethargy, sleepiness, dyspnea, possible coma, markedly decreased bone marrow activity, and RBC hemolysis** |
| Sudden massive entrapment of cells in spleen and liver ➡ | **Lethargy, pallor, and hypovolemic shock** |

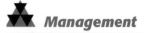 *Management*

♦ Copious amounts of oral or I.V. fluids — *to correct hypovolemia and prevent dehydration and vessel occlusion*
♦ Packed RBC transfusion — *to correct anemia or hypovolemia (if hemoglobin levels decrease)*
♦ Sedation and analgesics — *for pain*
♦ Oxygen administration — *to correct hypoxia*
♦ Ventilatory assistance — *for respiratory failure*
♦ Hydroxyurea — *to reduce painful episodes by increasing production of fetal hemoglobin*
♦ Iron and folic acid supplements — *to prevent megeloblastic anemia*
♦ Prophylactic penicillin (after age 2 months) — *to prevent infection*

# 13

# Fluid, electrolyte, and acid-base disorders

## Pathophysiologic concepts 312

## Disorders 314

# PATHOPHYSIOLOGIC CONCEPTS

## *Acidosis*

◆ Systemic increase in hydrogen ion concentration
◆ Occurs when:
– lungs fail to eliminate $CO_2$
– volatile (carbonic) or nonvolatile (lactic) acid products of metabolism accumulate
– hydrogen ion concentration rises
– persistent diarrhea causes loss of basic bicarbonate anions
– kidneys fail to reabsorb bicarbonate or secrete hydrogen ions

## *Alkalosis*

◆ Systemic decrease in hydrogen ion concentration
◆ Decreased hydrogen ion concentration may result from:
– excessive loss of $CO_2$ during hyperventilation
– loss of nonvolatile acids during vomiting
– excessive ingestion of base

## *Edema*

◆ Increased volume of fluid in interstitial spaces; results from abnormal expansion of interstitial fluid or accumulation of fluid in third spaces
◆ May be localized; caused by obstruction of veins or lymphatic system or by increased vascular permeability
◆ May be systemic (generalized); due to heart failure or renal disease
◆ Anasarca: massive systemic edema

## *Electrolyte imbalances*

◆ Too much or too little of any electrolyte will affect most body systems
◆ Insufficient or excess potassium, or insufficient calcium or magnesium, can increase excitability of cardiac muscle, causing arrhythmias
◆ Insufficient or excessive sodium or excess potassium can cause oliguria
◆ GI tract is particularly susceptible to electrolyte imbalance
  – excess potassium: abdominal cramps, nausea, and diarrhea
  – insufficient potassium: paralytic ileus
  – excess magnesium: nausea, vomiting, and diarrhea
  – excess calcium: nausea, vomiting, and constipation

## *Tonicity*

◆ Relative concentration of electrolytes (osmotic pressure) on both sides of semipermeable membrane (cell wall or capillary wall)
◆ Isotonic alterations: intracellular and extracellular fluids have equal osmotic pressure; dramatic change in total-body fluid volume occurs
◆ Hypertonic alterations: extracellular fluid is more concentrated than intracellular fluid; causes water to flow out of cell through semipermeable cell membrane (cell shrinkage)
◆ Hypotonic alterations: osmotic pressure forces some extracellular fluid into cells, causing cells to swell

# DISORDERS

## Hypovolemia

◆ Extracellular fluid volume deficit
◆ Characterized by isotonic loss of body fluids and relatively equal losses of sodium and water

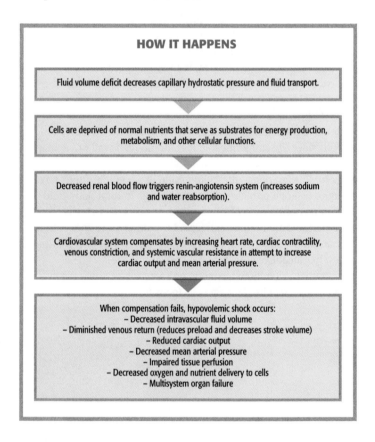

**HOW IT HAPPENS**

Fluid volume deficit decreases capillary hydrostatic pressure and fluid transport.

Cells are deprived of normal nutrients that serve as substrates for energy production, metabolism, and other cellular functions.

Decreased renal blood flow triggers renin-angiotensin system (increases sodium and water reabsorption).

Cardiovascular system compensates by increasing heart rate, cardiac contractility, venous constriction, and systemic vascular resistance in attempt to increase cardiac output and mean arterial pressure.

When compensation fails, hypovolemic shock occurs:
– Decreased intravascular fluid volume
– Diminished venous return (reduces preload and decreases stroke volume)
– Reduced cardiac output
– Decreased mean arterial pressure
– Impaired tissue perfusion
– Decreased oxygen and nutrient delivery to cells
– Multisystem organ failure

## *Causes*

- Excessive fluid loss
  - hemorrhage
  - excessive perspiration
  - renal failure (with polyuria)
  - abdominal surgery, fistulas
  - vomiting, diarrhea, nasogastric drainage
  - diabetes mellitus (with polyuria) or diabetes insipidus
  - excessive use of laxatives or diuretic therapy
  - fever
- Reduced fluid intake (dysphagia, coma, environmental conditions preventing fluid intake, or psychiatric illness)
- Third-spacing fluid shift
  - burns (during initial phase)
  - acute intestinal obstruction
  - acute peritonitis
  - pancreatitis
  - crushing injury
  - pleural effusion
  - hip fracture

## ▲ *Pathophysiologic changes*

| | |
|---|---|
| Decreased cardiac output ➡ | **Orthostatic hypotension, flattened neck veins** |
| Sympathetic nervous system response to increased cardiac output and mean arterial pressure ➡ | **Tachycardia** |
| Increased osmolality of extracellular fluid (stimulates thirst center in hypothalamus) ➡ | **Thirst** |
| Decreased volume of total-body fluids and dehydration of connective tissues and aqueous humor ➡ | **Sunken eyeballs, dry mucous membranes, diminished skin turgor** |
| Acute loss of body fluid ➡ | **Rapid weight loss** |
| Decreased renal perfusion from renal vasoconstriction ➡ | **Decreased urine output** |
| Increased systemic vascular resistance ➡ | **Prolonged capillary refill time** |

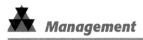 *Management*

---

- ◆ Oral fluids — *to treat mild hypovolemia (if patient is alert and can swallow)*
- ◆ Parenteral fluids — *to supplement or replace oral therapy*
- ◆ Fluid resuscitation by rapid I.V. administration (depending on patient's condition, 100 to 500 ml of fluid over 15 minutes to 1 hour; fluid bolus may be given more quickly if needed in severe fluid loss) — *to restore intravascular volume and raise blood pressure*
- ◆ Blood or blood products (with hemorrhage) — *to restore intravascular volume due to blood loss*
- ◆ Antidiarrheals (as needed) — *for diarrhea*
- ◆ Antiemetics (as needed) — *for vomiting*
- ◆ I.V. dopamine (Intropin) or norepinephrine (Levophed) — *to increase cardiac contractility and renal perfusion (if patient still symptomatic after fluid replacement)*
- ◆ Oxygen therapy — *to ensure sufficient tissue perfusion*
- ◆ Autotransfusion — *for hypovolemia caused by trauma*

---

# Hypervolemia

◆ Expansion of extracellular fluid volume; may involve interstitial or intravascular space
◆ Develops when excess sodium and water are retained in relatively same proportions
◆ Always secondary to increase in total-body sodium content

---

### HOW IT HAPPENS

Increased extracellular fluid volume (in interstitial or intravascular compartments)

Circulatory overload
Increased cardiac contractility and mean arterial pressure
Increased capillary hydrostatic pressure
Shift of fluid to interstitial space
Edema

With severe or prolonged hypervolemia or history of cardiovascular dysfunction:
Failure of compensatory mechanisms
Heart failure and pulmonary edema

---

## *Causes*

◆ Conditions that increase risk for sodium and water retention:
  – heart failure
  – cirrhosis of the liver (nephrotic syndrome)
  – corticosteroid therapy
  – low dietary protein intake
  – renal failure
◆ Excessive sodium and water intake:
  – parenteral fluid replacement with normal saline or lactated Ringer's solution
  – blood or plasma replacement
  – dietary intake of water, sodium chloride, or other salts
◆ Fluid shift to extracellular fluid compartment:
  – emobilization of fluid after burn treatment
  – hypertonic fluids (mannitol [Osmitrol])
  – hypertonic saline solution
  – colloid oncotic fluids (albumin)

## ◣ *Pathophysiologic changes*

Fewer red blood cells per milli-
liter of blood ▶        **Rapid breathing**

Increased fluid volume in pleural
spaces ▶        **Dyspnea**

Elevated hydrostatic pressure in
pulmonary capillaries ▶        **Crackles**

Increased cardiac contrac-
tility ▶        **Rapid, bounding pulse**

Increases in blood volume and
preload ▶        **Hypertension (unless heart is
failing), jugular vein distention**

Increased volume of total-body
fluid from circulatory overload
(best indicator of extracellular
fluid volume excess) ▶        **Acute weight gain**

Increased mean arterial pressure
leading to increased capillary hydrostatic pressure (causes fluid
shift from plasma to interstitial
spaces) ▶        **Edema**

Rapid filling and ventricular volume overload ▶        **S$_3$ gallop**

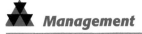

# Management

- Restricted sodium and water intake — *to prevent heart failure and pulmonary edema*
- Diuretics (furosemide) — *to promote fluid loss*
- Morphine, furosemide, and nitroglycerin (Nitro-Bid) — *to reduce preload in pulmonary edema*
- Hydralazine (Apresoline) and captopril (Capoten) — *to reduce afterload*
- Hemodialysis, continuous renal replacement therapy, or peritoneal dialysis — *for severe hypervolemia or renal failure*
- Oxygen administration — *to increase oxygen content of blood and tissues*

# Hyponatremia

◆ Serum sodium less than 135 mEq/L
◆ Characterized by diluted body fluids and cellular edema from decreased extracellular fluid osmolality
◆ If severe, can lead to seizures, coma, and permanent neurologic damage

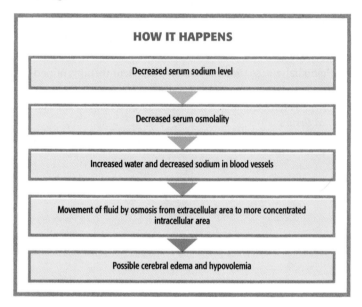

**HOW IT HAPPENS**

Decreased serum sodium level

Decreased serum osmolality

Increased water and decreased sodium in blood vessels

Movement of fluid by osmosis from extracellular area to more concentrated intracellular area

Possible cerebral edema and hypovolemia

## *Causes*

◆ Excessive sodium loss caused by GI losses, excessive sweating, burns, adrenal insufficiency, diuretic use, or starvation
◆ Dilutional hyponatremia from excessive water gain may result from:
   – increased administration of I.V. fluids
   – syndrome of inappropriate antidiuretic hormone
   – oxytocin use during labor
   – water intoxication
   – heart failure

# ▲ *Pathophysiologic changes*

| | |
|---|---|
| Osmotic swelling of cells ▶ | Muscle twitching and weakness |
| Altered neurotransmission ▶ | Lethargy, confusion, seizures, and coma |
| Decreased extracellular circulating volume ▶ | Hypotension and tachycardia |
| Edema affecting receptors in brain or vomiting center of brain stem ▶ | Nausea, vomiting, and abdominal cramps |
| Renal dysfunction ▶ | Oliguria or anuria |

# ▲ *Management*

- Restricted fluid intake and administration of oral sodium supplements — *to treat mild hyponatremia associated with hypervolemia*
- Isotonic I.V. fluids (normal saline solution) — *for hyponatremia associated with hypovolemia*
- High-sodium foods (if able to tolerate oral feedings) — *when serum sodium levels are below 110 mEq/L*
- Infusion of hypertonic (3% or 5% saline) solution slowly and in small volumes — *to prevent fluid overload*
- Administration of loop diuretics (furosemide) — *to increase water elimination*
- Monitoring for signs of circulatory overload or worsening neurologic status — *to prevent complications or promptly treat them if they occur*

# Hypernatremia

- ◆ Serum sodium greater than 145 mEq/L
- ◆ Characterized by excess sodium relative to body water
- ◆ If severe, can lead to seizures, coma, and permanent neurologic damage

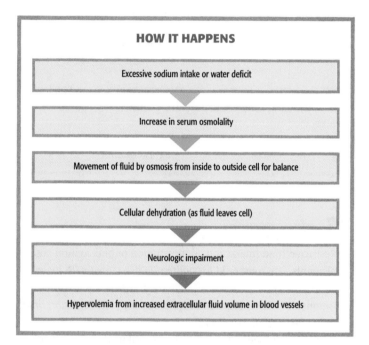

**HOW IT HAPPENS**

Excessive sodium intake or water deficit

↓

Increase in serum osmolality

↓

Movement of fluid by osmosis from inside to outside cell for balance

↓

Cellular dehydration (as fluid leaves cell)

↓

Neurologic impairment

↓

Hypervolemia from increased extracellular fluid volume in blood vessels

## *Causes*

- ◆ Water loss that exceeds sodium loss (profuse sweating, diarrhea, and polyuria)
- ◆ Sodium gain that exceeds water gain (salt intoxication)
- ◆ Hyperaldosteronism
- ◆ Use of diuretics, corticosteroids, or vasopressin

# 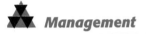 *Pathophysiologic changes*

Altered cellular metabolism ➡    Agitation, restlessness, fever, and decreased level of consciousness

Shifting of fluid from intracellular to intracellular space ➡    Hypertension, tachycardia, pitting edema, and excessive weight gain; thirst, increased viscosity of saliva, and rough tongue

Dramatic increase in osmotic pressure ➡    Dyspnea, respiratory arrest, and death

# ▲▲ *Management*

◆ Oral fluid replacement (gradually over 48 hours) — *to avoid shifting fluid into brain cells and to prevent cerebral edema*
◆ I.V. fluid replacement with salt-free solutions (dextrose 5% in water) — *to return sodium level to normal*
◆ Follow-up of I.V. infusion of half-normal saline solution — *to prevent hyponatremia and cerebral edema*
◆ Restricted oral sodium intake and use of diuretics with oral or I.V. fluid replacement — *to promote sodium loss*

# Hypokalemia

◆ Serum potassium less than 3.5 mEq/L
◆ Potassium deficiency caused by body's inability to effectively conserve potassium

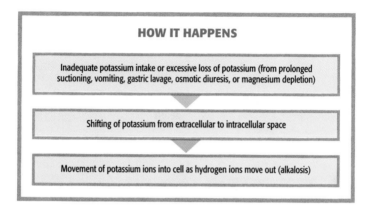

**HOW IT HAPPENS**

Inadequate potassium intake or excessive loss of potassium (from prolonged suctioning, vomiting, gastric lavage, osmotic diuresis, or magnesium depletion)

Shifting of potassium from extracellular to intracellular space

Movement of potassium ions into cell as hydrogen ions move out (alkalosis)

## *Causes*

◆ Loss of potassium in GI system (diarrhea, laxative abuse, prolonged vomiting or gastric suctioning, ileostomy, or colostomy)
◆ Loss of potassium in renal system (from diuretic therapy, diuretic phase of renal failure, or hyperaldosteronism)
◆ Steroid therapy
◆ Inadequate dietary intake of potassium (oral or parenteral nutrition)
◆ Alkalosis
◆ Treatment of diabetic ketoacidosis with insulin therapy

# ▲ *Pathophysiologic changes*

| | |
|---|---|
| Changes in membrane excitability ➡ | Dizziness, hypotension, arrhythmias, electrocardiogram (ECG) changes, and cardiac arrest |
| Decreased bowel motility ➡ | Nausea, vomiting, anorexia, diarrhea, decreased peristalsis, and abdominal distention |
| Decreased neuromuscular excitability ➡ | Muscle weakness, fatigue, and leg cramps |

# ▲▲ *Management*

- ◆ High-potassium diet — *to treat potassium deficit*
- ◆ Oral potassium supplements — *to treat potassium deficit*
- ◆ I.V. potassium — *for rapid replacement or inability to tolerate oral potassium supplements*

# Hyperkalemia

◆ Serum potassium greater than 5 mEq/L
◆ Characterized by excess potassium relative to body fluid; most dangerous electrolyte disorder
◆ Slight increase in potassium level can have profound consequences on neuromuscular and cardiovascular systems

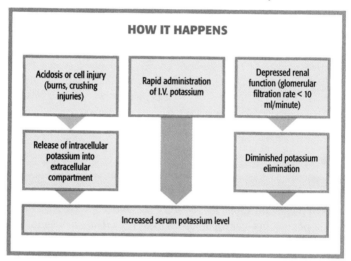

**HOW IT HAPPENS**

Acidosis or cell injury (burns, crushing injuries) → Release of intracellular potassium into extracellular compartment

Rapid administration of I.V. potassium

Depressed renal function (glomerular filtration rate < 10 ml/minute) → Diminished potassium elimination

Increased serum potassium level

## *Causes*

◆ Decreased renal excretion (oliguric renal failure, potassium-sparing diuretic therapy, or adrenal insufficiency)
◆ High potassium intake (excessive oral supplementation, excessive use of salt substitute, or rapid infusion of potassium solutions)
◆ Acidosis, tissue damage, or burns

# ▲ *Pathophysiologic changes*

| | |
|---|---|
| Altered repolarization ➡ | Tachycardia changing to brady-cardia, ECG changes, and cardiac arrest |
| Decreased gastric motility ➡ | Nausea, diarrhea, and abdominal cramps |
| Inactivation of membrane sodium channels ➡ | Muscle weakness and flaccid paralysis |

# ▲ *Management*

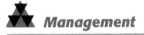

- ◆ Restricted potassium intake — *to decrease potassium intake or absorption*
- ◆ Medication evaluation and adjustment — *to eliminate or readjust medications that may be contributing to elevated potassium levels*
- ◆ Polystyrene sulfonate (Kayexalate) orally, via nasogastric tube, or as enema — *to exchange sodium ions for potassium ions in the intestine*
- ◆ Regular insulin and I.V. hypertonic dextrose — *to move potassium into cells and monitor for hypoglycemia*
- ◆ Sodium bicarbonate (in cases of acidosis) — *to shift potassium into cells*
- ◆ Calcium gluconate (10% solution) — *to counteract myocardial effects of hyperkalemia*

# Hypochloremia

♦ Serum chloride less than 98 mEq/L
♦ Characterized by deficiency of chloride in extracellular fluid
♦ Decreased serum chloride levels may affect levels of sodium, potassium, calcium, and other electrolytes (commonly associated with hyponatremia)

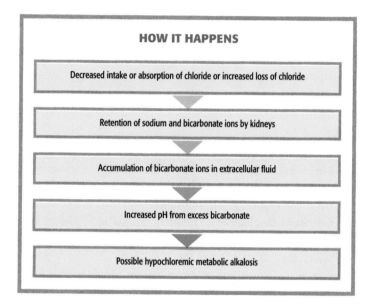

**HOW IT HAPPENS**

Decreased intake or absorption of chloride or increased loss of chloride

↓

Retention of sodium and bicarbonate ions by kidneys

↓

Accumulation of bicarbonate ions in extracellular fluid

↓

Increased pH from excess bicarbonate

↓

Possible hypochloremic metabolic alkalosis

## *Causes*

♦ Loss of chloride in GI system (excessive diarrhea, vomiting, or nasogastric suction)
♦ Diuretic therapy
♦ Diabetic ketoacidosis
♦ Burns

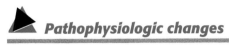

# Pathophysiologic changes

| | |
|---|---|
| Hyponatremia (usually occurs with hypochloremia) 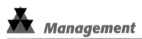 | Muscle weakness and twitching |
| Decreased serum chloride level ▶ | Metabolic alkalosis, tremors, and CNS hyperexcitability |

# Management

- Increased dietary intake of chloride, fluid administration (I.V. normal saline solution), or drug therapy — *to replace chloride loss*
- Treatment of associated metabolic alkalosis or electrolyte imbalances — *to correct abnormalities*

# Hyperchloremia

◆ Serum chloride greater than 108 mEq/L
◆ Characterized by excess chloride in extracellular fluid
◆ Typically associated with other acid-base imbalances; rarely occurs alone

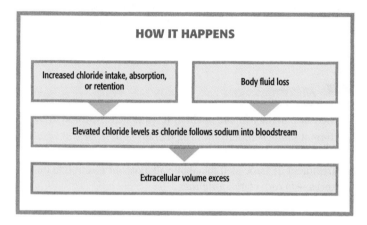

**HOW IT HAPPENS**

Increased chloride intake, absorption, or retention

Body fluid loss

Elevated chloride levels as chloride follows sodium into bloodstream

Extracellular volume excess

## *Causes*

◆ Dehydration
◆ Cushing syndrome
◆ Salicylate use

## ▲ *Pathophysiologic changes*

| | |
|---|---|
| Metabolic acidosis ➡ | Deep, rapid breathing (Kussmaul's respirations), weakness, and diminished cognitive ability (possibly leading to coma) |
| Extracellular fluid volume excess ➡ | Agitation, tachycardia, hypertension, pitting edema, dyspnea |

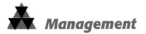

## Management

- Restriction of sodium and chloride — *to reduce chloride intake*
- Diuretic therapy (if not dehydrated) — *to eliminate chloride*
- Fluid administration (if dehydrated) — *to dilute chloride and force renal excretion*
- I.V. sodium bicarbonate (in severe hyperchloremia) — *to increase serum bicarbonate levels*

# Hypocalcemia

◆ Serum calcium less than 8.5 mg/dl; ionized serum calcium less than 4.5 mg/dl
◆ Occurs when calcium levels fall below normal range

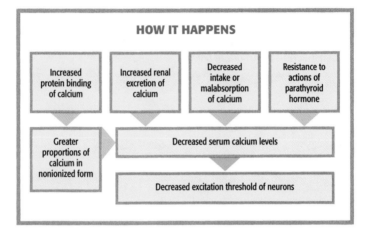

## Causes

◆ Hypoparathyroidism
◆ Infusion of citrated blood
◆ Acute pancreatitis
◆ Hyperphosphatemia
◆ Inadequate intake of calcium and vitamin D
◆ Magnesium deficiency
◆ Use of aminoglycosides, calcitonin, or corticosteroids
◆ Long-term laxative use

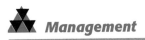

## Pathophysiologic changes

| | |
|---|---|
| Enhanced neuromuscular irritability ▶ | Anxiety, irritability, mouth twitching, laryngospasm, seizures, tetany, and positive Chvostek's and Trousseau's signs |
| Decreased calcium influx ▶ | Hypotension, ECG changes, and arrhythmias |

## Management

- ◆ Immediate calcium replacement with administration of I.V. calcium gluconate or calcium chloride — *for acute hypocalcemia*
- ◆ Magnesium replacement — *to enhance calcium therapy (hypocalcemia does not respond to calcium therapy alone)*
- ◆ Vitamin D supplementation (in chronic cases) — *to facilitate calcium absorption*
- ◆ Dietary adjustments — *to increase intake of calcium, vitamin D, and protein*
- ◆ Phosphate binders — *to lower elevated phosphorus levels (if necessary)*

# Hypercalcemia

- ◆ Serum calcium greater than 10.5 mg/dl; ionized serum calcium greater than 5.1 mg/dl
- ◆ Characterized as increase in total serum or ionized calcium level

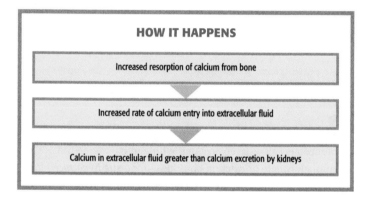

**HOW IT HAPPENS**

Increased resorption of calcium from bone

Increased rate of calcium entry into extracellular fluid

Calcium in extracellular fluid greater than calcium excretion by kidneys

## *Causes*

- ◆ Hyperparathyroidism and malignant neoplasms (major causes)
- ◆ Increased calcium intake
- ◆ Thiazide diuretic use
- ◆ Multiple fractures and prolonged immobility

# ◢ *Pathophysiologic changes*

| | |
|---|---|
| Decreased neuromuscular irritability (increased threshold) ➡ | Drowsiness, lethargy, headaches, irritability, confusion, depression, apathy, heart block |
| Depressed neuromuscular irritability and release of acetylcholine at myoneural junction ➡ | Weakness and muscle flaccidity |
| Calcium loss from bone ➡ | Bone pain and pathological fractures |
| Hyperosmolarity ➡ | Anorexia, nausea, vomiting, constipation, and dehydration |
| Kidney stone formation ➡ | Flank pain |

# ◣◥ *Management*

- ◆ Limited dietary intake of calcium — *to avoid excess levels*
- ◆ Discontinuation of medications or infusions containing calcium — *to lower calcium levels*
- ◆ Hydration (with normal saline solution) — *to prevent volume depletion, encourage diuresis, and increase urinary excretion of calcium*
- ◆ Loop diuretics — *to promote calcium excretion*
- ◆ Dialysis (if condition is life-threatening) — *to remove excess calcium*
- ◆ Corticosteroids — *to block bone resorption of calcium and decrease absorption in GI tract*
- ◆ Etidronate disodium — *to inhibit action of osteoclasts in bone*
- ◆ Mithramycin — *for hypercalcemia resulting from cancer*
- ◆ Calcitonin — *to inhibit bone resorption (effects are short-lived)*

# Hypomagnesemia

◆ Serum magnesium less than 1.5 mEq/L
◆ Occurs when magnesium serum level is low
◆ Typically accompanied by hypokalemia and hypocalcemia

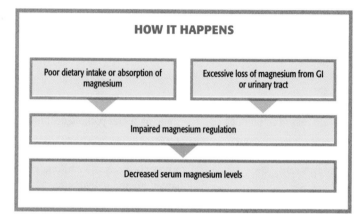

**HOW IT HAPPENS**

| Poor dietary intake or absorption of magnesium | Excessive loss of magnesium from GI or urinary tract |

Impaired magnesium regulation

Decreased serum magnesium levels

## *Causes*

◆ Alcoholism
◆ Protein-calorie malnutrition
◆ Diarrhea or gastric suctioning
◆ Malabsorption syndrome, intestinal bypass
◆ Anorexia, bulimia
◆ Hyperaldosteronism
◆ Use of osmotic diuretics or antibiotics
◆ Burns, sepsis, pancreatitis
◆ Exchange transfusion

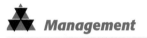 *Pathophysiologic changes*

| | |
|---|---|
| Altered neuromuscular transmission ➡ | Hyperirritability, tetany, leg and foot cramps, positive Chvostek's and Trousseau's signs, confusion, delusions, and seizures |
| Enhanced inward sodium current or concurrent effects of calcium and potassium imbalance ➡ | Arrhythmias, vasodilation, and hypotension |

## ▲▲▲ *Management*

- ◆ Dietary replacement or oral magnesium supplements (in mild cases) — *to replace magnesium (takes several days)*
- ◆ I.V. or I.M. doses of magnesium sulfate (in severe cases) — *to replenish depleted magnesium (requires careful assessment of renal function)*

# Hypermagnesemia

◆ Serum magnesium greater than 2.5 mEq/L
◆ Uncommon condition resulting from decreased renal excretion (renal failure) or increased intake of magnesium

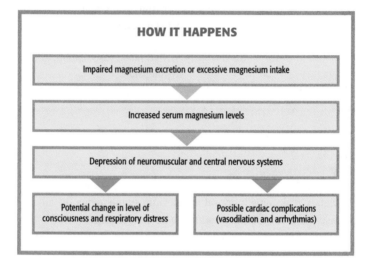

**HOW IT HAPPENS**

Impaired magnesium excretion or excessive magnesium intake

↓

Increased serum magnesium levels

↓

Depression of neuromuscular and central nervous systems

↓

Potential change in level of consciousness and respiratory distress

Possible cardiac complications (vasodilation and arrhythmias)

## *Causes*

◆ Renal failure
◆ Excessive antacid use
◆ Adrenal insufficiency
◆ Excessive magnesium replacement or excessive use of milk of magnesia or other magnesium-containing laxatives

# ▲ *Pathophysiologic changes*

| | |
|---|---|
| Suppressed release of acetylcholine at myoneural junction (blocks neuromuscular transmission and reduces cell excitability) ▶ | **Diminished reflexes, muscle weakness, or flaccid paralysis** |
| Respiratory muscle paralysis ▶ | **Respiratory distress** |
| Decreased inward sodium current ▶ | **Heart block, bradycardia** |
| Relaxation of vascular smooth muscle and reduction of vascular resistance (by displacing calcium from vascular wall surface) ▶ | **Hypotension** |

# ▲ *Management*

- ◆ Oral or I.V. fluids (with normal renal function) — *to rid body of excessive magnesium*
- ◆ Loop diuretics (if increased fluids unsuccessful) — *to promote magnesium excretion*
- ◆ Calcium gluconate (magnesium antagonist) — *for relief of symptoms in an emergency*
- ◆ Mechanical ventilation (if levels are toxic) — *to treat respiratory distress*
- ◆ Hemodialysis with magnesium-free dialysate solution — *for severe renal dysfunction or if excess magnesium can't be eliminated*
- ◆ Withdrawal of magnesium-containing medications and restricted dietary intake of magnesium — *to lower magnesium level*

# Hypophosphatemia

◆ Serum phosphate less than 2.5 mg/dl
◆ Indicates deficiency of phosphorus, but can occur under circumstances when total body phosphorus stores are normal
◆ Considered severe when serum levels are less than 1 mg/dl; can lead to organ failure

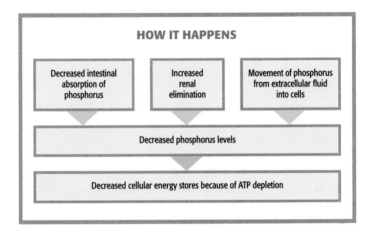

**HOW IT HAPPENS**

Decreased intestinal absorption of phosphorus

Increased renal elimination

Movement of phosphorus from extracellular fluid into cells

Decreased phosphorus levels

Decreased cellular energy stores because of ATP depletion

## *Causes*

◆ Malabsorption syndromes, diarrhea, vomiting
◆ Alcoholism
◆ Prolonged glucose administration (orally or parenterally) resulting in insulin release
◆ Diabetic ketoacidosis
◆ Starvation
◆ Diuretic therapy or use of drugs that bind with phosphate (aluminum hydroxide)

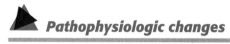 *Pathophysiologic changes*

| | |
|---|---|
| Deficiency of adenosine triphosphate (ATP) 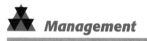 | Muscle weakness, tremor, and paresthesia |
| 2,3-diphosphoglycerate deficiency ➡ | Peripheral hypoxia |

 *Management*

- ◆ Diet high in phosphorus and use of oral phosphorus supplements — *to treat moderate hypophosphatemia*
- ◆ I.V. replacement with potassium phosphate or sodium phosphate (in severe cases) — *to replenish phosphorus level*
- ◆ Careful monitoring for "refeeding syndrome" (in patient starting total parenteral nutrition) — *to control shift of phosphorus into cell (usually occurs 3 or more days after feedings begin)*

# Hyperphosphatemia

♦ Serum phosphate greater than 4.5 mg/dl
♦ Occurs when kidneys are unable to excrete excess phosphorus and serum levels rise
♦ Usually asymptomatic unless condition leads to hypocalcemia

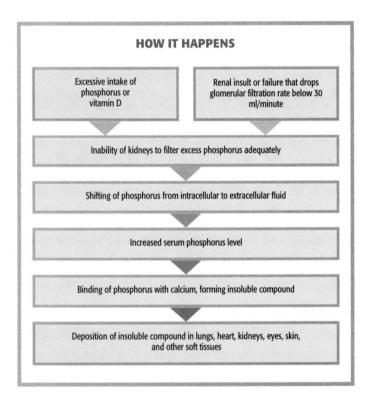

**HOW IT HAPPENS**

| Excessive intake of phosphorus or vitamin D | Renal insult or failure that drops glomerular filtration rate below 30 ml/minute |

Inability of kidneys to filter excess phosphorus adequately

Shifting of phosphorus from intracellular to extracellular fluid

Increased serum phosphorus level

Binding of phosphorus with calcium, forming insoluble compound

Deposition of insoluble compound in lungs, heart, kidneys, eyes, skin, and other soft tissues

## *Causes*

♦ Renal disease
♦ Hypoparathyroidism
♦ Massive trauma, muscle necrosis
♦ Excessive phosphate intake

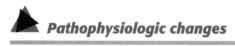

## Pathophysiologic changes

| | |
|---|---|
| Enhanced neuromuscular irritability ▶ | Irritability, anxiety, mouth twitching, laryngospasm, tetany, positive Chvostek's and Trousseau's signs |
| Decreased calcium influx ▶ | Hypotension, ECG changes, and arrhythmias |

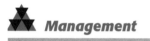

## Management

♦ Limited dietary intake of phosphorus or use of phosphorus-containing medications — *to decrease phosphorus levels*
♦ Use of aluminum, magnesium, or calcium gel or phosphate binding agents — *to decrease absorption of phosphorus in GI system*
♦ Administration of I.V. saline solution (in severe cases) — *to promote renal excretion (ineffective in patients with renal insufficiency)*
♦ Dialysis — *to reduce phosphate levels if hyperphosphatemia is related to renal failure*

# Metabolic acidosis

◆ Acid-base imbalance characterized by excess acid and deficient $HCO_3^-$
◆ Caused by underlying nonrespiratory disorder
◆ Primary decrease in plasma $HCO_3^-$ causes pH to fall
◆ Can occur with:
  – increased production of nonvolatile acid (lactic acid)
  – decreased renal clearance of nonvolatile acid (renal failure)
  – loss of $HCO_3^-$ (chronic diarrhea)
◆ Symptoms result from action of compensatory mechanisms in lungs, kidneys, and cells
◆ Prognosis improves with prompt treatment of underlying cause and rapid reversal of acidotic state

**THE PATHO PICTURE**

## UNDERSTANDING METABOLIC ACIDOSIS

This series of illustrations shows how metabolic acidosis develops at the cellular level.

**Step 1**

As hydrogen ions (H) start to accumulate in the body, chemical buffers in the cells and extracellular fluid bind with them.

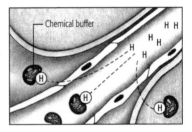

**Step 2**

Excess hydrogen ions that the buffers can't bind with decrease the pH and stimulate chemoreceptors in the medulla to increase the respiratory rate. The increased respiratory rate lowers the $PaCO_2$, which allows more hydrogen ions to bind with bicarbonate ions ($HCO_3^-$).

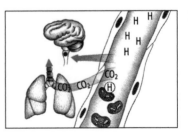

### Step 3

Healthy kidneys try to compensate for acidosis by secreting excess hydrogen ions into the renal tubules.

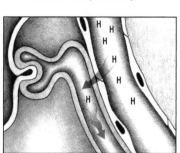

### Step 4

Each time a hydrogen ion is secreted into the renal tubules, a sodium ion (Na) and a bicarbonate ion are absorbed from the tubules and returned to the blood.

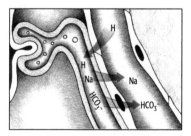

### Step 5

Excess hydrogen ions in the extracellular fluid diffuse into cells. To maintain the balance of the charge across the membrane, the cells release potassium ions (K) into the blood.

### Step 6

Excess hydrogen ions alter the normal balance of potassium, sodium, and calcium ions (Ca), leading to reduced excitability of nerve cells.

## *Causes*

- ◆ Excessive production of metabolic acids: diabetic ketoacidosis, lactic acidosis, malnutrition, starvation, chronic alcoholism
- ◆ Excessive bicarbonate loss: GI loss (diarrhea, intestinal suction) and renal loss (renal failure, hyperaldosteronism)
- ◆ Other causes: salicylate intoxication, exogenous poisoning, decreased tissue oxygenation or perfusion

### *Pathophysiologic changes*

| | |
|---|---|
| Change in pH level ▶ | **Headache, malaise, and lethargy progressing to drowsiness** |
| Change in electrolyte balance from excess hydrogen ion (results in impaired neural excitability) ▶ | **CNS depression** |
| Compensatory mechanism of lungs to blow off $CO_2$ ▶ | **Kussmaul's respirations** |
| Decreased cardiac output resulting from increasing pH ▶ | **Hypotension** |
| GI distress ▶ | **Anorexia, nausea, vomiting, diarrhea, and possible dehydration** |
| pH-sensitive decrease in vascular response to sympathetic stimuli ▶ | **Warm, flushed skin** |

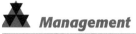

## *Management*

◆ Sodium bicarbonate I.V. (for severe high anion gap in patients with pH less than 7.20 and $HCO_3^-$ loss) — *to neutralize blood acidity*

◆ Monitoring of plasma electrolytes (especially potassium) during sodium bicarbonate therapy (potassium level may fall as pH rises) — *to prevent or treat imbalances*

◆ I.V. fluids — *to correct normal anion gap metabolic acidosis and extracellular fluid volume deficit*

◆ Mechanical ventilation (if needed) — *to maintain respiratory compensation*

◆ Antibiotics — *to treat infection*

◆ Dialysis — *to treat renal failure or certain drug toxicities*

◆ Antidiarrheal agents — *to treat diarrhea-induced $HCO_3^-$ loss*

# Metabolic alkalosis

◆ Acid-base imbalance characterized by decreased amounts of acid and increased amounts of base bicarbonate
◆ Occurs when low levels of acid or high $HCO_3^-$ cause metabolic, respiratory, and renal responses
◆ Occurs secondary to underlying cause

**THE PATHO PICTURE**

## UNDERSTANDING METABOLIC ALKALOSIS

This series of illustrations shows, at the cellular level, how metabolic alkalosis develops.

**Step 1**

As bicarbonate ions ($HCO_3^-$) start to accumulate in the body, chemical buffers bind with the ions.

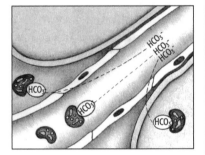

**Step 2**

Excess bicarbonate ions that don't bind with chemical buffers elevate serum pH levels, which in turn depress chemoreceptors in the medulla. Depression of those chemorecptors causes a decease in respiratory rate, which increases the $Paco_2$. The additional $CO_2$ combines with water to form carbonic acid ($H_2CO_3$).

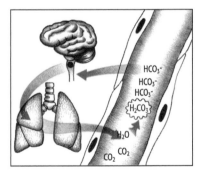

**UNDERSTANDING METABOLIC ALKALOSIS** *(continued)*

### Step 3

When the bicarbonate level exceeds 28 mEq/L, the renal glomeruli can no longer reabsorb excess bicarbonate. That excess bicarbonate is excreted in the urine; hydrogen ions are retained.

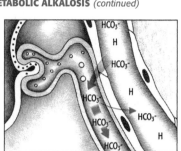

### Step 4

To maintain electrochemical balance, the kidneys excrete excess sodium ions (Na), water, and bicarbonate.

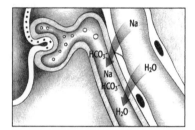

### Step 5

Lowered hydrogen ion levels in the extracellular fluid cause the ions to diffuse out of the cells. To maintain the balance of charge across the cell membrane, extracellular potassium ions (K) move into the cells.

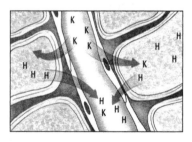

### Step 6

As hydrogen ion levels decline, calcium (Ca) ionization decreases. That decrease in ionization makes nerve cells more permeable to sodium ions. Sodium ions moving into nerve cells stimulate neural impulses and produce overexcitability of the peripheral and central nervous systems.

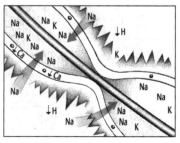

## *Causes*

◆ Loss of acid, retention of base, or renal mechanisms associated with low serum levels of potassium and chloride
◆ Critical acid loss:
  – chronic vomiting
  – nasogastric tube drainage or lavage without adequate electrolyte replacement
  – fistulas
  – use of steroids and certain diuretics (furosemide, thiazides, ethacrynic acid)
  – massive blood transfusions
  – Cushing's disease, primary hyperaldosteronism, and Bartter's syndrome
◆ Excessive $HCO_3^-$ retention (causes chronic hypercapnia):
  – excessive intake of bicarbonate of soda or other antacids or absorbable alkali
  – excessive amounts of I.V. fluids with high concentrations of bicarbonate or lactate
  – alterations in extracellular electrolyte levels
  – low plasma potassium, causing increased hydrogen ion excretion by kidneys

## ▲ *Pathophysiologic changes*

| | |
|---|---|
| Decreased cerebral perfusion ▶ | **Irritability, picking at bedclothes (carphology), twitching, confusion** |
| Hypokalemia ▶ | **Arrhythmias** |
| Compensatory response when severe respiratory alkalosis leads to respiratory failure ▶ | **Slow, shallow respirations** |
| Diminished peripheral blood flow (during repeated blood pressure checks) ▶ | **Carpopedal spasm in hand (Trousseau's sign, possible sign of impending tetany)** |

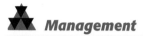

## Management

♦ Potassium chloride and normal saline solution (except in heart failure) — *to replace losses from gastric drainage*
♦ Discontinuation of diuretics and supplementary potassium chloride — *to prevent further electrolyte loss*
♦ Oral or I.V. acetazolamide — *to enhance renal bicarbonate excretion and correct metabolic alkalosis without rapid volume expansion*

# Respiratory acidosis

◆ Acid-base imbalance characterized by reduced alveolar ventilation

◆ Caused by inability of pulmonary system to clear enough $CO_2$ from body

◆ Leads to hypercapnia ($Paco_2$ greater than 45 mm Hg) and acidosis (pH less than 7.35)

◆ May be acute (sudden failure in ventilation) or chronic (long-term pulmonary disease)

---

**THE PATHO PICTURE**

### UNDERSTANDING RESPIRATORY ACIDOSIS

This series of illustrations shows how respiratory acidosis develops at the cellular level.

**Step 1**

When pulmonary ventilation decreases, retained carbon dioxide ($CO_2$) combines with water ($H_2O$) to form carbonic acid ($H_2CO_3$). The carbonic acid dissociates to release free hydrogen ions (H) and bicarbonate ions ($HCO_3^-$). The excessive carbonic acid causes a drop in pH.

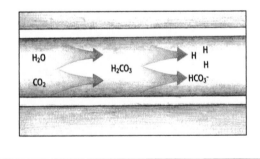

**UNDERSTANDING RESPIRATORY ACIDOSIS** *(continued)*

## Step 2

As the pH level falls, 2,3-diphosphoglycerate (2,3,-DPG) increases in the red blood cells and causes a change in hemoglobin (Hb) that makes the hemoglobin release oxygen ($O_2$). The altered hemoglobin, now strongly alkaline, picks up hydrogen ions and $CO_2$, thus eliminating some of the free hydrogen ions and excess $CO_2$.

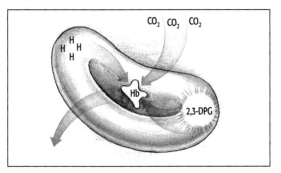

## Step 3

Whenever $Pa_{CO_2}$ increases, $CO_2$ builds up in all tissues and fluids. The $CO_2$ reacts with water to form carbonic acid, which then breaks into free hydrogen ions and bicarbonate ions. The increased amount of $CO_2$ and free hydrogen ions stimulate the respiratory center to increase the respiratory rate. An increased respiratory rate expels more $O_2$ and helps reduce the $CO_2$ level in the blood and other tissues.

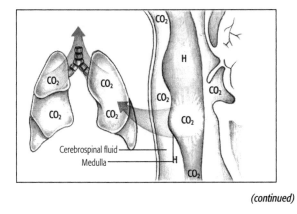

*(continued)*

**UNDERSTANDING RESPIRATORY ACIDOSIS** *(continued)*

**Step 4**

$CO_2$ and hydrogen ions cause cerebral blood vessels to dilate, which increases blood flow to the brain.

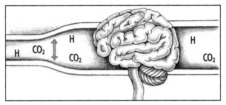

**Step 5**

As respiratory mechanisms fail, the increasing $Paco_2$ stimulates the kidneys to conserve bicarbonate and sodium ions and to excrete hydrogen ions, some as ammonium ($NH_4$). The additional bicarbonate and sodium combine to form extra sodium bicarbonate ($NaHCO_3$), which is then able to buffer more free hydrogen ions.

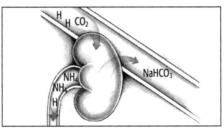

**Step 6**

As the concentration of hydrogen ions overwhelms the body's compensatory mechanisms, the hydrogen ions move into the cells and potassium ions move out. A concurrent lack of oxygen causes an increase in the anaerobic production of lactic acid, which further skews the acid-base balance.

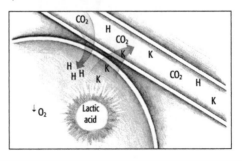

## Causes

◆ Drugs that decrease sensitivity of respiratory center (narcotics, general anesthetics, hypnotics, alcohol, sedatives)
◆ Central nervous system trauma (injury to medulla may impair ventilatory drive)
◆ Cardiac arrest
◆ Sleep apnea
◆ Chronic metabolic alkalosis
◆ Ventilation therapy:
  – high positive end-expiratory pressure with reduced cardiac output (may cause hypercapnia)
  – neuromuscular diseases (myasthenia gravis, Guillain-Barré syndrome, poliomyelitis); respiratory muscles can't respond properly to respiratory drive
  – airway obstruction, acute respiratory distress syndrome, chronic obstructive pulmonary disease, asthma
  – large pneumothorax, extensive pneumonia, pulmonary edema

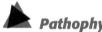 *Pathophysiologic changes*

Cerebral edema and depressed central nervous system activity (from dilation of cerebral blood vessels and increased blood flow to brain) ➡ Restlessness, confusion, apprehension, somnolence, fine or flapping tremor (asterixis), coma, headaches; dyspnea and tachypnea; papilledema; depressed reflexes; hypoxemia (unless patient is receiving oxygen); tachycardia, atrial and ventricular arrhythmias; hypertension; hypotension with vasodilation (bounding pulses and warm periphery, in severe acidosis)

# ▲▲▲ *Management*

◆ Correction of underlying cause — *to improve alveolar ventilation*
◆ Insertion of artificial airway (endotracheal intubation or tracheotomy), mechanical ventilation, oxygen therapy — *to maintain adequate ventilation*
◆ Increase of partial pressure of arterial oxygen ($Pao_2$) to at least 60 mm Hg and pH greater than 7.2 — *to prevent cardiac arrhythmias*
◆ Aerosolized or I.V. bronchodilators — *to open constricted airways*
◆ Positive end-expiratory pressure — *to prevent alveolar collapse*
◆ Bronchoscopy — *to remove excessive retained secretions*

# Respiratory alkalosis

◆ Acid-base imbalance characterized by $Paco_2$ less than 35 mm Hg and blood pH greater than 7.45

◆ Caused by alveolar hyperventilation

◆ Hypocapnia occurs when lungs eliminate more $CO_2$ than cells produce

**THE PATHO PICTURE**

## UNDERSTANDING RESPIRATORY ALKALOSIS

This series of illustrations shows how respiratory alkalosis develops at the cellular level.

**Step 1**

When pulmonary ventilation increases above the amount needed to maintain normal carbon dioxide ($CO_2$) levels, excessive amounts of CO2 are exhaled. This causes hypocapnia (a fall in $PaCO_2$), which leads to a reduction in carbonic acid ($H2CO_3$) production, a loss of hydrogen (H) ions and bicarbonate ions ($HCO_3$-), and a subsequent rise in pH.

**Step 2**

Hydrogen ions are pulled out of the cells and into the blood in exchange for potassium ions (K). The hydrogen ions entering the blood combine with bicarbonate ions to form carbonic acid, which lowers the pH.

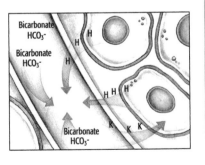

*(continued)*

**UNDERSTANDING RESPIRATORY ALKALOSIS** (continued)

**Step 3**
Hypocapnia stimulates the carotid and aortic bodies and the medulla, which causes an increase in heart rate without an increase in blood pressure.

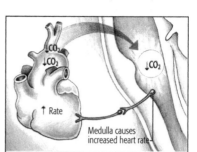

**Step 4**
Hypocapnia produces cerebral vasoconstriction, which prompts a reduction in cerebral blood flow. Hypocapnia also overexcites the medulla, pons, and other parts of the autonomic nervous system.

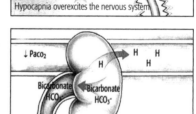

Decreased $Paco_2$ causes vasoconstriction

$\downarrow Paco_2$

Hypocapnia overexcites the nervous system

**Step 5**
When hypocapnia lasts more than 6 hours, the kidneys increase secretion of bicarbonate and reduce excretion of hydrogen.

$\downarrow Paco_2$

H   H
H      H

Bicarbonate $HCO_3^-$   Bicarbonate $HCO_3^-$

**Step 6**
Continued low $Paco_2$ increases cerebral and peripheral hypoxia from vasoconstriction. Severe alkalosis inhibits calcium (Ca) ionization, which in turn causes increased nerve excitability and muscle contractions.

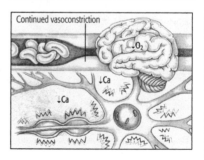

Continued vasoconstriction

$\downarrow O_2$

$\downarrow Ca$

$\downarrow Ca$

## *Causes*

◆ Pulmonary-related: severe hypoxemia, pneumonia, interstitial
lung disease, pulmonary vascular disease, acute asthma
◆ Nonpulmonary-related: anxiety, fever, aspirin toxicity, metabolic acidosis, central nervous system disease (inflammation or
tumor), sepsis, hepatic failure, pregnancy

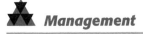

## *Pathophysiologic changes*

| | |
|---|---|
| Hypoxemia ➡ | Cardinal signs: deep, rapid breathing (greater than 40 breaths/minute; much like Kussmaul's respirations in diabetic acidosis) |
| Decreased cerebral blood flow and CNS excitability ➡ | Light-headedness or dizziness, agitation; circumoral and peripheral paresthesias; carpopedal spasms, twitching (can progress to tetany), muscle weakness |

## *Management*

◆ Correction of underlying cause — *to reduce alveolar hyperventilation*
◆ Oxygen — *for acute hypoxemia*
◆ Breathing into paper bag — *to increase $CO_2$ level and relieve hyperventilation caused by severe anxiety*
◆ Adjustment of tidal volume and minute ventilation — *to prevent hyperventilation*

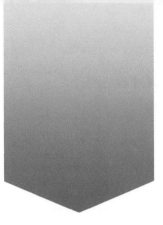

**Additional disorders: A quick review**

**Selected references**

**Index**

# Additional disorders:
# A quick review

| Pathophysiology | Signs and symptoms |
|---|---|

### Adenoid hyperplasia
Enlargement of lymphoid tissue of nasopharynx resulting from increased mitosis, which leads to increased number of cells in adenoid tissue. May be hereditary or due to chronic infections.

◆ Respiratory obstruction (mouth breathing; snoring at night; frequent, prolonged nasal congestion)
◆ Persistent mouth breathing (during formative years)
◆ Sinusitis, frequent otitis media

### Adrenogenital syndrome
Excessive adrenal androgen production that causes somatic masculinization, virilization, and hermaphrodism. Lack of enzyme needed to synthesize cortisol causes excessive ACTH response through negative feedback loop to pituitary, sending continual ACTH message to adrenal glands and resulting in hyperplasia of adrenal tissue. Excessive androgen production is stimulated because adrenal pathway to androgen production is not blocked.

◆ Enlarged external genitalia in newborn due to excessive androgen production (female infants may have slightly enlarged clitoris or clitoris with penile shape and fused labia resembling scrotum; males have enlarged genitals)
◆ Severe electrolyte imbalance, dehydration, vomiting, wasting, and shock due to adrenal crisis (at 5 to 10 days)

### Albinism
Absence of enzyme tyrosine results in a defect in melanin formation, resulting in partial or total lack of melanin pigment.

◆ Extremely fair skin color
◆ Fine, white hair
◆ Gray or blue irises of eye
◆ Strabismus, nystagmus, photophobia
◆ Persistent loss of visual acuity

### Alpha$_1$-antitrypsin deficiency
Reduced or absent levels of alpha$_1$-antitrypsin (needed to inhibit proteolytic enzymes) leads to unopposed action of protease on liver and lungs.

*In children:*
◆ Cholestasis
◆ Hepatitis
◆ Portal hypertension
*In young adults:*
◆ Emphysema
◆ Cirrhosis

| Pathophysiology | Signs and symptoms |
|---|---|
| **_Amblyopia_** <br> Reduced acuity resulting from toxic reaction in orbital portion of optic nerve or cerebral blockage of visual stimuli. | ◆ Visual dimness, photophobia, ocular discomfort <br> ◆ Small central or pericentral scotoma that enlarges slowly <br> ◆ Temporal disk pallor <br> ◆ Possible blindness |
| **_Amyloidosis_** <br> Rare, chronic disease of abnormal fibrillar scleroprotein (waxy, starchlike glycoprotein) accumulation that infiltrates body organs and soft tissues. Perireticular type affects inner coats of blood vessels; pericollagen type affects outer coats. Amyloidosis can result in permanent, even life-threatening, organ damage. | ◆ Proteinuria, leading to nephrotic syndrome and eventually renal failure <br> ◆ Heart failure (due to cardiomegaly); arrhythmias; amyloid deposits in subendocardium, endocardium, and myocardium <br> ◆ Tongue stiffness and enlargement, decreased intestinal motility, malabsorption, bleeding, abdominal pain, constipation, diarrhea <br> ◆ Peripheral neuropathy <br> ◆ Liver enlargement (possibly with azotemia, anemia, albuminuria, and jaundice) |
| **_Ankylosing spondylitis_** <br> Infiltration of fibrous tissue of joint capsule by inflammatory cells that erode bone and fibrocartilage. Repair of cartilaginous structures begins with proliferation of fibroblasts, which synthesize and secrete collagen; collagen formation produces fibrous scar tissue that eventually undergoes calcification and ossification, causing joint to fuse or lose flexibility. | ◆ Intermittent low back pain (most severe following inactivity or in morning) <br> ◆ Stiffness, limited lumbar spine motion <br> ◆ Chest pain, limited chest expansion <br> ◆ Peripheral arthritis (shoulders, hips, knees) <br> ◆ Kyphosis (in advanced stages) <br> ◆ Hip deformity, limited range of motion <br> ◆ Mild fatigue, fever, and anorexia or weight loss <br> ◆ Dyspnea (if costovertebral joints are involved) |

| Pathophysiology | Signs and symptoms |
|---|---|
| ***Aspergillosis***<br>Fungal infection caused by *Aspergillus,* which produces extracellular enzymes (proteases and peptidases) that contribute to tissue invasion, leading to hemorrhage and necrosis. | ◆ Incubation (few days to weeks): may be asymptomatic or mimic tuberculosis, causing productive cough and purulent or blood-tinged sputum, dyspnea, empyema, and lung abscesses<br>◆ Allergic aspergillosis: wheezing, dyspnea, pleural pain, and fever<br>◆ Aspergillosis endophthalmitis (appears 2 to 3 weeks after eye surgery): cloudy vision, eye pain, reddened conjunctiva, and purulent exudates |
| ***Behçet's syndrome***<br>Sudden inflammation of small blood vessels caused by overactive immune system; symptoms based on inflammation site. Most common in those of Mediterranean, Middle Eastern, and Far Eastern descent. Onset is usually ages 10 to 20; five times more common in males. | ◆ Recurrent genital and oral ulcerations, skin lesions<br>◆ Eye inflammation<br>◆ Subcutaneous thrombophlebitis, deep vein thrombosis<br>◆ Epididymitis<br>◆ Arterial occlusion and aneurysm<br>◆ Severe headache, fatigue<br>◆ Bloating, diarrhea, cramping, bloody stools<br>◆ Movement and speech difficulties |
| ***Blastomycosis***<br>Fungal infection caused by *Blastomyces dermatitidis.* Inhalation of conidia leads to clearing of organism by alveolar macrophages; those conidia not destroyed convert to yeast forms that trigger inflammatory response, resulting in formation of noncaseating granulomas. | ◆ Dry, hacking, or productive cough<br>◆ Pleuritic chest pain, dyspnea<br>◆ Fever, tremor, chills, night sweats, malaise, anorexia<br>◆ Small, painless, nonpruritic, and nondistinctive macules or papules on exposed body parts<br>◆ Painful swelling of testes, epididymis, or prostate; deep perineal pain, pyuria, and hematuria |

| Pathophysiology | Signs and symptoms |
|---|---|
| ***Bronchiectasis***<br>Inflammation and destruction of structural components of bronchial wall that leads to chronic abnormal dilation. | *In early stages:*<br>◆ Asymptomatic (may complain of frequent pneumonia or hemoptysis)<br>◆ Chronic cough producing copious, foul-smelling, mucopurulent secretions and hemoptysis<br>◆ Coarse crackles during inspiration<br>◆ Wheezing, dyspnea, sinusitis, fever, chills<br>*In advanced stage:*<br>◆ Chronic malnutrition and right-sided heart failure due to hypoxic pulmonary vasoconstriction |
| ***Bronchiolitis***<br>Acute infection resulting from necrosis of bronchial epithelium and destruction of ciliated epithelial cells. As submucosa becomes edematous, cellular debris and fibrin form plugs in bronchioles. | *Subacute symptoms:*<br>◆ Fever, persistent nonproductive cough, dyspnea, malaise, and anorexia<br>◆ Dry crackles<br>*Less common:*<br>◆ Tachypnea, tachycardia, intercostal and subcostal retractions<br>◆ Productive cough, hemoptysis, chest pain, general aches, night sweat |
| ***Brucellosis***<br>Acute febrile illness caused by nonmotile, nonspore-forming, gram-negative coccobacilli of *Brucella* species. | *In acute phase:*<br>◆ Fever, chills, profuse sweating, fatigue, headache, backache, enlarged lymph nodes<br>◆ Anorexia, joint pain, enlarged spleen<br>*In chronic phase:*<br>◆ Depression, sleep disturbances, sexual impotence |

| Pathophysiology | Signs and symptoms |
| --- | --- |

### Celiac disease

Bowel disorder resulting from inability to hydrolyze peptides contained in gluten. Ingestion of gluten causes injury to villi in upper small intestine, leading to decreased surface area and malabsorption of most nutrients. Causes inflammatory enteritis, osmotic diarrhea, and secretory diarrhea.

◆ Recurrent diarrhea, abdominal distention, stomach cramps, weakness, muscle wasting, increased appetite without weight gain
◆ Normochromic, hypochromic, or macrocytic anemia
◆ Osteomalacia, osteoporosis, tetany, bone pain in lower back, rib cage, or pelvis
◆ Peripheral neuropathy, paresthesia, seizures
◆ Dry skin, eczema, psoriasis, dermatitis herpetiformis, acne rosacea
◆ Amenorrhea, hypometabolism, adrenocortical insufficiency
◆ Extreme lethargy, mood swings, irritability

### Cervical cancer

Preinvasive cancer (curable with early detection) causes minimal cervical dysplasia in lower third of epithelium; invasive cancer penetrates basement membrane to disseminate throughout body via lymphatic routes. Histologic type is 95% squamous cell carcinoma.

*Preinvasive cancer:*
◆ Abnormal vaginal bleeding, persistent vaginal discharge
◆ Postcoital pain and bleeding
*Advanced stages:*
◆ Pelvic pain
◆ Vaginal leakage of urine or feces due to fistula
◆ Anorexia, weight loss, anemia

### Cervical spondylosis

Condition caused by progressive myelopathy, resulting in cord compression and spastic gait.

◆ Pain or loss of feeling in affected arm and shoulder, stiffness of cervical spine
◆ Arm weakness and atrophy with reflex loss
◆ Hyperreflexia, increased muscle tone
◆ Plantar extensor response in legs

### Chalazion

Blockage of meibomian gland that leads to formation of granulation tissue.

◆ Local swelling, mild irritation
◆ Blurred vision
◆ Red-yellow elevation on conjunctival surface under eyelid

| Pathophysiology | Signs and symptoms |
|---|---|
| **Chédiak-Higashi syndrome**<br>Genetic defect that manifests in morphologic changes in granulocytes and causes delayed chemotaxis and impaired intracellular digestion of organisms; diminished inflammatory response results. | ◆ Recurrent bacterial infections (skin, lungs, subcutaneous tissue)<br>◆ Fever, significant photophobia<br>◆ Thrombocytopenia, neutropenia, hepatosplenomegaly<br>◆ Motor and sensory neuropathies<br>◆ Cellular proliferation of liver, spleen, and bone marrow (fatal) |
| **Cholera**<br>Acute GI infection caused by colonization of small intestine following ingestion of a significant inoculum. Secretion of potent enterotoxin results in massive outpouring of isotonic fluid from mucosal surface of small intestine. Profuse diarrhea, vomiting, and fluid and electrolyte loss occur; may lead to hypovolemic shock, metabolic acidosis, and death. | ◆ Following incubation period (several hours to 5 days): acute, painless, profuse watery diarrhea, and vomiting<br>◆ Intense thirst, weakness, loss of skin tone; dehydration; electrolyte imbalances; oliguria<br>◆ Muscle cramps<br>◆ Cyanosis<br>◆ Tachycardia<br>◆ Falling blood pressure, fever, and hypoactive bowel sounds |
| **Chronic fatigue and immune dysfunction syndrome**<br>Condition characterized by abnormal immune response and hormonal alterations as result of infectious agents or environmental factors. | ◆ Constellation of symptoms: myalgia, arthralgia with arthritis, low-grade fever, pain, cervical adenopathy, sore throat, headache, memory deficits, sleep disturbances<br>◆ Prolonged, overwhelming fatigue |
| **Coccidioidomycosis**<br>Fungal infection caused by *Coccidioides immitis,* resulting in granulomatous reaction and caseous necrosis. | ◆ Dry cough, pleuritic chest pain, dyspnea, pleural effusion<br>◆ Fever, sore throat, chills, malaise, headache<br>◆ Itchy macular rash<br>◆ Tender red nodules on legs with joint pain in knees and ankles (Caucasian women)<br>◆ Chronic pulmonary cavitation<br>◆ Anorexia, weight loss |

| Pathophysiology | Signs and symptoms |
|---|---|
| **Colorado tick fever**<br>Vector-borne virus that circulates inside erythropoietic cells, producing typical febrile symptoms. | ◆ Immediately following incubation (3 to 6 days): chills, high fever, lethargy, severe back, arm, and leg aches<br>◆ Headache with ocular movement<br>◆ Photophobia, abdominal pain, nausea, vomiting |
| **Common variable immunodeficiency**<br>Condition characterized by progressive deterioration of B-cell (humoral) immunity. Most patients have a normal circulating B-cell count, but have defective synthesis or release of immunoglobulins. Many also exhibit progressive deterioration of T-cell (cell-mediated) immunity revealed by delayed hypersensitivity skin testing. | ◆ Initial symptoms: recurrent sinopulmonary infections, chronic bacterial conjunctivitis, and malabsorption<br>◆ Chronic pyogenic bacterial infections |
| **Complement deficiencies**<br>Series of circulating enzymatic serum proteins with nine functional components labeled C1-C9. Deficiencies may increase susceptibility to infections and certain autoimmune disorders. | *C5 deficiency (familial defect in infants):*<br>◆ Diarrhea, seborrheic dermatitis<br>*C1 esterase inhibitor deficiency:*<br>◆ Swelling in face, hands, abdomen, or throat<br>◆ Laryngeal edema (may be fatal)<br>*C2 and C3 deficiencies and C5 familial dysfunction:*<br>◆ Increased susceptibility to bacterial infection<br>*C2 and C4 deficiencies:*<br>◆ Collagen vascular disease (lupus and chronic renal failure) |
| **Costochondritis**<br>Inflammatory process of costochondral or costosternal joints that causes localized pain and tenderness. | ◆ Sharp pain in chest wall<br>◆ Area sensitive to touch<br>◆ Pain radiating into arm<br>◆ Pain worsening with movement<br>◆ Reproducible pain |

| Pathophysiology | Signs and symptoms |
|---|---|
| **Creutzfeldt-Jakob disease**<br>Rare, fatal brain disorder that infects central nervous system, leading to myelin destruction and neuronal loss. | ◆ Myoclonic jerking, ataxia, aphasia, visual disturbances, paralysis, early abnormal electroencephalogram<br>◆ Possible dementia |
| **Croup**<br>Acute childhood disease caused by viral infection and characterized by inflammation and spasms of upper airway, resulting in severe larynx constriction and reduced airflow. Inflammatory changes almost completely obstruct larynx (which includes the epiglottis) and significantly narrow the trachea. | ◆ Inspiratory stridor, hoarse or muffled vocal sounds, varying degrees of laryngeal obstruction and respiratory distress<br>◆ Characteristic sharp, barking, seallike cough<br>◆ With progression: inflammatory edema and possible spasms (may obstruct upper airway and severely compromise ventilation) |
| **Cryptococcosis**<br>Asymptomatic pulmonary infection that disseminates to extrapulmonary sites (usually central nervous system but also skin, bones, prostate gland, liver, or kidneys). Untreated, infection progresses from coma to death due to cerebral edema or hydrocephalus. | ◆ Fever, cough with pleuritic pain, weight loss<br>◆ Severe frontal and temporal headache, diplopia, blurred vision, dizziness, aphasia, vomiting<br>◆ Skin abscesses and painful lesions of long bones, skull, spine, and joints |
| **Cystic echinococcosis**<br>Infection of tapeworm larvae *(Echinococcus)* characterized by cyst formation. *E. granulosus* forms cysts in liver, lungs, kidneys, and spleen; infection can be treated with surgery. *E. multilocularis* (alveolar hydatid disease) forms parasite tumors in liver, lungs, brain, and other organs; infection can be fatal. | ◆ Slow-growing cysts (may be asymptomatic for years; symptoms depend on location and size of cysts) |
| **Cystinuria**<br>Inherited disease characterized by impaired function of membrane-carrier proteins essential for transport of cystine and other dibasic amino acids, resulting in excessive amino acid concentration in urine and excessive urinary excretion of cystine. | ◆ Dull flank pain and capsular distention from acute renal colic<br>◆ Hematuria<br>◆ Tenderness in costovertebral angle or over kidneys<br>◆ Urinary obstruction with secondary infection (fever, chills, frequency, foul-smelling urine) |

| Pathophysiology | Signs and symptoms |
|---|---|

### DiGeorge syndrome

Congenital condition in which abnormal fetal development of third and fourth pharyngeal pouches interferes with thymus formation. Thymus is absent or partially present in abnormal site, causing deficient cell-mediated immunity. Without fetal thymus transplant, results in death by age 2.

◆ Appearance at birth: low-set ears, notches in ear pinna, fish-shaped mouth, undersized jaw, abnormally wide-set eyes
◆ Great vessel anomalies, tetralogy of Fallot
◆ Hypocalcemia
◆ Early heart failure

### Encephalitis

Intense lymphocytic infiltration of brain tissues and leptomeninges resulting from viral infection. Causes cerebral edema, degeneration of brain's ganglion cells, and diffuse nerve cell destruction.

◆ Acute stage: sudden onset of fever, headache, and vomiting
◆ Meningeal irritation (stiff neck and back), neuronal damage (drowsiness, coma, paralysis, seizures, ataxia, tremors, nausea, vomiting, organic psychoses)
◆ Possible coma (may persist for days or weeks)

### Epicondylitis

Inflammation of extensor tendons of forearm or flexor muscles of wrist, probably resulting from partial tear at affected site. Untreated, may become disabling as adherent fibers form between tendons and elbow capsule.

◆ Elbow pain (gradually worsens, usually radiates to forearm and back of hand when grasping object or twisting elbow)
◆ Tenderness over involved lateral or medial epicondyle or over head of radius
◆ Weak grasp

### Epidermolysis bullosa

Group of disorders (mostly inherited) characterized by appearance of vesicles and bullae caused by frictional trauma or heat. Prognosis depends on severity; often fatal in infancy and childhood, but becomes less severe as patient matures.

◆ Vesicles and bullae (on hands, feet, knees, or elbows as well as in GI, respiratory, or genitourinary tracts)
◆ Eyelid blisters, conjunctivitis, adhesions, corneal opacities
◆ Skin sloughing (large areas on newborn)
◆ Scars and contractures (possible with healing)

| Pathophysiology | Signs and symptoms |
| --- | --- |

### Epiglottiditis

Acute inflammation of epiglottis, sometimes preceded by upper respiratory infection, which may rapidly progress to complete upper airway obstruction within 2 to 5 hours. Laryngeal obstruction results from inflammation and edema.

◆ High fever, stridor, sore throat, dysphagia, irritability, restlessness, drooling
◆ Posturing (hyperextending neck, sitting up, leaning forward with mouth open, tongue protruding, and nostrils flaring to relieve respiratory distress)
◆ Inspiratory retractions, rhonchi

### Esophageal varices

Shunting of blood to venae cavae due to portal hypertension, which leads to complex of enlarged, swollen, and tortuous veins at lower end of the esophagus.

◆ Hemorrhage, hypotension
◆ Altered level of consciousness
◆ Hematemesis

### Fanconi's syndrome

Inherited disorder marked by changes in proximal renal tubules due to atrophy of epithelial cells and loss of proximal tube volume, resulting in shortened connection to glomeruli by unusually narrow segment. Malfunction of proximal renal tubules leads to hyperkalemia, hypernatremia, glycosuria, phosphaturia, aminoaciduria, uricosuria, acidosis, retarded growth, and rickets.

◆ At birth: generally normal appearance, slightly low birth weight
◆ After 6 months: weakness, failure to thrive, dehydration, cystine crystals in corners of eye, retinal pigment degeneration
◆ Yellowed skin with little pigmentation
◆ Slow linear growth

### Galactosemia

Inherited defect characterized by inability to metabolize galactose. Galactose-1-phosphate and galactose accumulate in tissues, leading to decreased hepatic output of glucose and hypoglycemia.

◆ Nausea, vomiting, diarrhea
◆ Jaundice, hepatomegaly
◆ Mental retardation, malnourishment, progressive hepatic failure, possible death

### Gallbladder and bile duct carcinoma

Rapidly growing, fatal cancer in which direct extension to liver, cystic and common bile ducts, stomach, and colon causes obstructions and consequent progressive, profound jaundice and epigastric and right upper quadrant pain.

◆ Ulcerative colitis (difficult to distinguish from cholecystitis)
◆ Pain in epigastrium or upper right quadrant
◆ Weight loss, anorexia, chills, fever
◆ Nausea, vomiting, jaundice
◆ Pruritus, skin excoriations

| **Pathophysiology** | **Signs and symptoms** |
| --- | --- |
| ***Gas gangrene***<br>Local infection in which bacteria produce hydrolytic enzymes and toxins that destroy connective tissue and cellular membranes, causing gas bubbles to form in muscle cells. Enzymes also lyse RBC membranes, destroying their oxygen-carrying capacity. | ◆ Myositis, soft-tissue anaerobic cellulitis<br>◆ Crepitus<br>◆ Severe localized pain, swelling<br>◆ Bullae, necrosis (after 36 hours)<br>◆ Ruptured wound (dark red or black necrotic muscle, foul-smelling watery or frothy discharge)<br>◆ Intravascular hemolysis, thrombosis, toxemia, hypovolemia<br>◆ Toxic delirium |
| ***Gastric cancer***<br>Increased nitrosoamine production that damages DNA of mucosal cells, promoting metaplasia and neoplasia. | ◆ Early stage: chronic dyspepsia, epigastric discomfort<br>◆ Late stage: weight loss, anorexia, fullness after eating, anemia, fatigue, dysphagia, vomiting, blood in stool |
| ***Gastritis***<br>Acute or chronic inflammation of gastric mucosa, which produces mucosal bleeding, edema, hemorrhage, and erosion. | ◆ Rapidly developing epigastric discomfort, indigestion, cramping, anorexia, nausea, vomiting, hematemesis |
| ***Giant cell arteritis***<br>Immune-related process in which lymphocytes, plasma cells, and multinucleated giant cells infiltrate affected vessels. Patchy or segmental changes overcome medium and large arteries of head and neck and may extend into carotids and aorta. Cell-mediated immune response directed toward antigens in or near elastic tissue component of arterial wall may account for this disorder. | ◆ Continuous throbbing, intractable temporal headache<br>◆ Ischemia of masseter muscles, tongue, and pharynx<br>◆ Scalp necrosis and ulceration<br>◆ Ocular or orbital pain<br>◆ Transient loss of vision, visual field defects, blurring, hallucinations<br>◆ Tender, red, swollen, and nodular temporal arteries with diminished pulses<br>◆ Sudden blindness<br>◆ Pale, swollen optic disk surrounded by pericapillary hemorrhage<br>◆ Chewing difficulty, weight loss, fever<br>◆ Depression |

| Pathophysiology | Signs and symptoms |
|---|---|

### Gilbert's disease
Genetic defect characterized by impaired hepatic bilirubin clearance that results in hyperbilirubinemia.

◆ Mild jaundice (without dark urine)
◆ Nausea, vomiting
◆ Portal hypertension, ascites, skin or endocrine changes
◆ Abdominal pain, anorexia, malaise

### Globoid cell leukodystrophy
Deficiency of galactosylceramidase leads to rapid cerebral demyelination with large globoid bodies in white matter and central nervous system.

◆ Irritability, rigidity, blindness, tonic-clonic seizures, deafness, mental deterioration

### Goodpasture's syndrome
Condition characterized by abnormal production of autoantibodies directed against alveolar and glomerular basement membranes, leading to immune-mediated inflammation of lung and kidney tissues.

◆ Cough, bloody sputum, dyspnea
◆ Anemia
◆ Peripheral edema
◆ Hematuria, elevated serum creatinine and protein levels, progressive renal failure

### Hand, foot, and mouth disease
Highly contagious childhood disease in which RNA virus produces fever and vesicles in oropharynx and on hands and feet.

◆ Painful vesicular lesions on mouth, tongue, hands, and feet

### Hemothorax
Blood in chest from damaged intercostal, pleural, mediastinal, and (infrequently) lung parenchymal vessels that enter pleural cavity. Depending on amount of bleeding and underlying cause, hemothorax may be associated with varying degrees of lung collapse and mediastinal shift. Commonly accompanied by pneumothorax.

◆ Chest pain, tachypnea, mild to severe dyspnea
◆ Marked blood loss, hypotension, shock
◆ Chest expansion and stiffening (affected side only)

| Pathophysiology | Signs and symptoms |
|---|---|
| **Hereditary hemorrhagic telangiectasia**<br>Dilation of venules and capillaries leading to formation of fragile masses of thin convoluted vessels (telangiectases), resulting in abnormal tendency to hemorrhage. | ◆ Localized clusters of dilated capillaries (on face, ears, scalp, hands, arms, and feet; under nails; on mucous membranes of nose, mouth, and stomach), causing frequent epistaxis, hemoptysis, and GI bleeding<br>◆ Characteristic appearance: violet, non-pulsatile vessels that may be flat or raised, bleed spontaneously, and blanch on pressure<br>◆ Generalized capillary fragility (spontaneous bleeding, petechiae, ecchymoses, spider hemangiomas of varying sizes; may exist without overt telangiectasia) |
| **Herpangina**<br>Acute infection in which RNA virus produces fever and vesicles in posterior portion of oropharynx. | ◆ Sore throat, pain with swallowing<br>◆ Fever (100° to 104° F [37.8° to 40° C]) lasting for 1 to 4 days, febrile seizures<br>◆ Anorexia, malaise, vomiting, diarrhea<br>◆ Gray-white papulovesicles on soft palate<br>◆ Headache<br>◆ Pain in abdomen, neck, and extremities |
| **Hiatal hernia**<br>Weakening of anchors from gastroesophageal junction to diaphragm or increased abdominal pressure that allows herniation of part of stomach through esophageal hiatus in diaphragm. | ◆ Reflux of gastric contents, indigestion (heartburn)<br>◆ Dysphagia<br>◆ Chest pain |
| **Hirsutism**<br>Androgen excess that causes signs of masculinization (abnormal hair growth and distribution in women), pituitary dysfunction (precocious puberty), and adrenal dysfunction (Cushing's syndrome). May be hereditary or result of endocrine dysfunction or pharmacologic effects (minoxidil, androgenic steroids, testosterone). | ◆ Excessive hair growth in women or children (typically in adult male distribution pattern) |

| **Pathophysiology** | **Signs and symptoms** |
|---|---|

### Hydronephrosis

Abnormal dilation of renal pelvis and calyces of one or both kidneys due to obstructed urine flow in genitourinary tract. Partial obstruction and hydronephrosis may not produce initial symptoms, but pressure built up behind area of obstruction results in symptomatic renal dysfunction. Total obstruction of urine flow with dilation of collecting system ultimately causes complete cortical atrophy and cessation of glomerular filtration.

◆ Mild pain, slightly decreased urinary flow
◆ Severe, colicky renal pain or dull flank pain (may radiate to groin), gross urinary abnormalities (hematuria, pyuria, dysuria, alternating oliguria and polyuria, or complete anuria)
◆ Nausea, vomiting, abdominal fullness
◆ Pain, dribbling, or hesitancy with urination; infection due to urinary stasis

### Hyperbilirubinemia

Massive destruction of red blood cells that causes high levels of bilirubin in blood.

◆ Elevated levels of serum bilirubin
◆ Jaundice

### Hypersplenism

Increased spleen activity where all types of blood cells are removed from circulation due to chronic myelogenous leukemia, lymphomas, Gaucher's disease, hairy cell leukemia, or sarcoidosis (also possibly portal hypertension, malaria, tuberculosis, and various connective tissue and inflammatory diseases). Spleen growth may be stimulated by increased workload, such as with trapping and destroying of abnormal red blood cells.

◆ Enlarged spleen
◆ Cytopenia
◆ Abdominal pain on left side
◆ Fullness after eating small amounts of food

### Idiopathic pulmonary fibrosis

Chronic, progressive lung disease associated with inflammation and fibrosis, possibly resulting from tuberculosis or pneumoconiosis. Interstitial inflammation consists of alveolar septal infiltrate of lymphocytes, plasma cells, and histiocytes. Fibrotic areas are composed of dense acellular collagen. Areas of honeycombing that form are composed of cystic fibrotic air spaces, frequently lined with bronchiolar epithelium and filled with mucus. Smooth muscle hyperplasia may occur in areas of fibrosis and honeycombing.

◆ Dyspnea
◆ Nonproductive cough
◆ Chest heaviness
◆ Wheezing
◆ Anorexia
◆ Weight loss

| **Pathophysiology** | **Signs and symptoms** |
|---|---|
| **Intussusception** Telescoping of bowel portion into adjacent distal portion, propelled along by peristalsis and resulting in edema, hemorrhage from venous engorgement, incarceration, and obstruction. If treatment is delayed for longer than 24 hours, strangulation of intestine usually occurs, causing gangrene, shock, and perforation. | ◆ Intermittent attacks of colicky pain<br>◆ Vomiting<br>◆ "Currant jelly" stools (contain mixture of blood and mucus)<br>◆ Abdominal tenderness and distention; palpable abdominal mass (sausage-shaped) |
| **Kaposi's sarcoma** Malignant AIDS-related cancer arising from vascular endothelial cells that affects endothelial tissue, which compromises all blood vessels. | ◆ Circular, red-purple or brown lesions (appear slightly raised on face, arms, neck, and legs)<br>◆ Internal lesions (especially in GI tract, identified by biopsy) |
| **Keratitis** Ulceration of cornea due to bacterial infection, trauma, or autoimmune disorders. | ◆ Decreased visual acuity<br>◆ Eye pain<br>◆ Photophobia |
| **Kidney cancer** Renal cell carcinoma that produces tumors of various cell types and patterns. Tumors are usually aggressive in growth and affect younger patients. | ◆ Hematuria, flank pain, increased erythrocyte sedimentation rate<br>◆ Palpable mass<br>◆ Weight loss, anemia, fever, hypertension |
| **Kyphosis** Excessive curvature of spine with convexity backward due to congenital anomaly, tuberculosis, syphilis, malignant or compression fracture, arthritis, or rickets. | ◆ Abnormally rounded thoracic curve<br>◆ Back pain (possible) |
| **Lassa fever** Epidemic hemorrhagic fever transmitted to humans by contact with rodent urine, feces, or saliva infected by *Lassa* species. | ◆ Fever lasting 2 to 3 weeks<br>◆ Exudative pharyngitis, oral ulcers, dysphagia, swelling of face and neck<br>◆ Lymphadenopathy<br>◆ Purpura, ecchymoses<br>◆ Conjunctivitis<br>◆ Bradycardia, shock, peripheral collapse<br>◆ Pleural effusion (with renal involvement) |

| Pathophysiology | Signs and symptoms |
|---|---|

### Legionnaires' disease
Acute bronchopneumonia produced by gram-negative bacillus. Transmission occurs with inhalation of organism carried in aerosols produced by air-conditioning units, water faucets, shower heads, humidifiers, and contaminated respiratory equipment.

- Dry cough
- Myalgia
- GI distress, diarrhea
- Pneumonia
- Cardiovascular collapse

### Leprosy
Chronic, systemic infection with progressive cutaneous lesions, attacking the peripheral nervous system.

- Skin lesions
- Anesthesia
- Muscle weakness
- Paralysis

### Listeriosis
Infection due to gram-positive bacillus *Listeria monocytogenes,* resulting in febrile illness. Transmitted to neonates in utero; also transmitted by inhalation, consumption, or contact with contaminated unpasteurized milk, infected animals, or contaminated sewage or soil.

- Fever, malaise, lethargy
- Meningitis
- Spontaneous abortion

### Mastocytosis
Proliferation of mast cells systemically and within skin.

- Urticaria pigmentosa, flushing
- Diarrhea, abdominal pain, ascites
- Headache, vascular collapse

### Mastoiditis
Inflammation and infection of air cells of mastoid antrum, usually as result of chronic otitis media.

- Dull ache and tenderness around mastoid process, facial paralysis, labyrinthitis
- Headache, low-grade fever
- Thick, purulent drainage
- Brain abscess, meningitis

### Medullary sponge kidney
Genetic disorder in which collecting ducts in renal pyramids dilate, forming cavities, clefts, and cysts that produce complications of calcium oxalate stones and infections.

- Renal calculi
- Hematuria
- Infection (fever, chills, malaise)

| **Pathophysiology** | **Signs and symptoms** |
| --- | --- |

### Melasma

Hypermelanotic skin disorder associated with increased hormonal levels with pregnancy, oral contraceptive use, and ovarian cancer. Thought to be due to effects of estrogen and progesterone on melanin production.

◆ Patchy, nonraised, hypermelanotic rash

### Multiple endocrine neoplasia

Hereditary disorder in which two or more endocrine glands develop hyperplasia, adenoma, or carcinoma. Multiple endocrine neoplasia (MEN) I (Werner's syndrome) involves hyperplasia and adenomatosis of pituitary and parathyroid glands, islet cells of pancreas and, rarely, thyroid and adrenal glands. MEN II (Sipple's syndrome) involves medullary carcinoma of thyroid, with hyperplasia and adenomatosis of adrenal medulla (pheochromocytoma) and parathyroid glands.

*MEN I:*
◆ Hyperparathyroidism, hypercalcemia
◆ Ulcer (Zollinger-Ellison syndrome)
◆ Hypoglycemia
*MEN II:*
◆ Enlarged thyroid mass, with increased calcitonin and possible ectopic corticotropin (Cushing's syndrome)
◆ Headache, tachyarrhythmias, and hypertension (adrenal medulla tumors)
◆ Renal calculi (adenomatosis or hyperplasia of parathyroids)

### Myelitis

Inflammation of spinal cord that can result from several diseases (measles, pneumonia, syphilis, acute disseminated encephalomyelitis, poliovirus, herpes) as well as certain toxic agents or smallpox or polio vaccination. May involve inflammation of cord's gray matter (producing motor dysfunction) or white matter (producing sensory dysfunction); these types of myelitis can attack any level of spinal cord, causing partial destruction or scattered lesions. Acute transverse myelitis, the most devastating form, has a rapid onset and affects entire thickness of spinal cord, producing motor and sensory dysfunction.

◆ Sensory or motor dysfunction (depends on site of damage to spinal cord)
◆ Acute transverse myelitis: rapid motor and sensory dysfunction below level of spinal cord damage (appears in 1 to 2 days); flaccid paralysis of legs with loss of sensory and sphincter function; disappearance of reflexes (may reappear later); possible shock (hypotension and hypothermia; may occur with severe spinal cord damage)

### Myelodysplastic syndromes

Preleukemic disorders that progress to leukemia, caused by genetic factors and exposure to chemicals or radiation.

◆ Pancytopenia, anemia
◆ Weakness, fatigue
◆ Palpitations
◆ Dizziness, irritability

| Pathophysiology | Signs and symptoms |
|---|---|

### Narcolepsy
Chronic, recurrent attacks of drowsiness and sleep during daytime, resulting from familial factors.

◆ Drowsiness, daytime sleepiness
◆ Sudden loss of muscle tone
◆ Extreme emotional lability

### Necrotizing enterocolitis
Diffuse or patchy intestinal necrosis, often accompanied by sepsis; most common in premature infants and those of low birth weight. May develop when infant suffers perinatal hypoxemia due to shunting of blood from gut to more vital organs. Subsequent mucosal ischemia provides ideal medium for bacterial growth. As bowel swells and breaks down, gas-forming bacteria invade damaged areas, producing free air in intestinal wall, sometimes resulting in fatal perforation and peritonitis.

◆ Distended (especially tense or rigid) abdomen with gastric retention
◆ Increasing residual gastric contents (may contain bile)
◆ Bile-stained vomitus
◆ Occult blood in stool
◆ Thermal instability, lethargy, metabolic acidosis, jaundice, disseminated intravascular coagulation

### Neurofibromatosis
Group of inherited developmental disorders of nervous system, muscles, bones, and skin that affects cell growth of neural tissue.

◆ Café-au-lait spots
◆ Multiple, pediculated, soft tumors (neurofibromas)
◆ Hearing loss
◆ Bone changes, skeletal deformities

### Neurogenic arthropathy
Progressive degenerative disease of peripheral and axial joints, resulting from impaired sensory innervation due to diabetes mellitus, tabes dorsalis, syringomyelia, myelopathy of pernicious anemia, spinal cord trauma, paraplegia, hereditary sensory neuropathy, or Charcot-Marie-Tooth disease. Loss of joint sensation causes progressive deterioration, resulting from trauma or primary disease, which leads to laxity of supporting ligaments and eventual disintegration of affected joints.

◆ Joint swelling, warmth, decreased mobility, and instability (may occur in one or more joints)
◆ Progressive deformity
◆ Joint pain (minimal despite deformity)

| Pathophysiology | Signs and symptoms |
|---|---|
| **_Orbital cellulitis_**<br>Inflammation and infection of fatty orbital tissues and eyelids due to streptococcal, staphylococcal, or pneumococcal organisms. | ◆ Unilateral eyelid edema<br>◆ Hyperemia<br>◆ Redden eyelids, matted lashes |
| **_Osgood-Schlatter disease_**<br>Painful, incomplete separation of epiphysis of tibial tubercle from tibial shaft. Most common in active adolescent boys; may result from trauma before complete fusion of epiphysis to main bone has occurred (between ages 10 and 15). Trauma may be single action or repeated knee flexion against tight quadriceps muscle. Severe disease may cause permanent tubercle enlargement. | ◆ Constant aching, pain, and tenderness below kneecap<br>◆ Obvious soft-tissue swelling, localized heat and tenderness |
| **_Pediculosis_**<br>Infestation of parasitic forms of lice anywhere on body, most commonly on scalp (pediculosis capitis). Louse attaches to hair shaft with claws and feeds on blood several times daily; resides close to scalp to maintain its body temperature. Itching may be due to allergic reaction to louse saliva or irritability. | ◆ Itching, inflammation<br>◆ Eczematous dermatitis<br>◆ Fatigue, irritability, weakness<br>◆ Lice or nits in hair (head, axilla, pubic area) |
| **_Penile cancer_**<br>Benign or malignant neoplasms of penis. Malignancies are usually squamous cell carcinomas. Preceded by chronic irritation, condyloma acuminatum, or phimosis in uncircumcised men. | ◆ Painless ulcerations on glans or foreskin; small, warty plaques<br>◆ Dysuria, urinary obstruction, purulent penile discharge |

| Pathophysiology | Signs and symptoms |
|---|---|

### Phenylketonuria

Disorder characterized by insufficient hepatic phenylalanine hydroxylase (enzyme that acts as catalyst in conversion of phenylalanine to tyrosine). As a result, phenylalanine and its metabolites accumulate in blood, causing mental retardation if left untreated. The exact mechanism that causes retardation is unclear.

◆ Signs of arrested brain development: mental retardation (usually evident by age 4 months), personality disturbances (schizoid and antisocial personality patterns, uncontrollable temper)
◆ Characteristic features: light complexion, blue eyes
◆ Microcephaly; eczematous skin lesions or dry, rough skin; musty (mousy) odor
◆ Abnormal EEG patterns, possible seizures

### Pheochromocytoma

Tumor of chromaffin cells of adrenal medulla that causes increased production of catecholamines.

◆ Hypertension, high blood glucose and lipid levels
◆ Headache, palpitations, sweating, dizziness, syncope, anxiety, constipation

### Pilonidal disease

Coccygeal cyst that forms in intergluteal cleft on posterior surface of lower sacrum. It usually contains hair and becomes infected, producing abscess, draining sinus, or fistula. It may develop congenitally or from hirsutism; also may develop from stretching or irritation of sacrococcygeal area from prolonged rough exercise, heat, excessive perspiration, or constricting clothing.

◆ Signs of infection: localized pain, tenderness, swelling, or heat at site; continuous or intermittent purulent drainage; abscess formation; chills, fever, headache, and malaise

### Pituitary tumor

Intracranial neoplasm, most commonly macroadenoma, with self-secreting thyroid-stimulating hormone. As pituitary adenomas grow, they replace normal glandular tissue and enlarge the sella turcica, which houses pituitary gland.

◆ Signs of hyperthyroidism (without skin and eye manifestations)
◆ Goiter
◆ High free-thyroxine levels

### Pleurisy

Inflammation of visceral and parietal pleurae that line inside of thoracic cage and envelop lungs. Common causes include lupus, rheumatoid arthritis, and tuberculosis.

◆ Sharp, stabbing chest pain
◆ Dyspnea
◆ Pleural friction rub

| Pathophysiology | Signs and symptoms |
|---|---|
| **Pneumoconioses** | |
| Chronic and permanent disposition of particles (usually dust in occupational setting) in lungs that causes tissue reaction, which may be harmless or destructive. | ◆ Emphysema<br>◆ Shortness of breath, cough<br>◆ Fatigue, weakness<br>◆ Weight loss |
| **Polycythemia vera** | |
| Chronic myeloproliferative disorder characterized by increased production of red blood cells, neutrophils, and platelets that inhibits blood flow to microcirculation, resulting in intravascular thrombosis. May result from multipotential stem cell defect. | *Early stage:*<br>◆ Absence of symptoms (symptoms appear later due to expanded blood volume within affected body system)<br>*Later stages:*<br>◆ Weakness, headache, light-headedness, vision disturbances, fatigue<br>◆ Hepatomegaly, splenomegaly<br>◆ Maroon or plum-color skin and mucous membranes<br>◆ Hypertension |
| **Polymyositis** | |
| Diffuse, inflammatory myopathy that produces symmetrical weakness of striated muscles (proximal muscles of shoulder, pelvic girdle, neck, and pharynx) via lymphocytic infiltration. | ◆ Proximal muscle weakness, dysphonia, dysphagia, and regurgitation<br>◆ Polyarthralgia, joint effusion, Raynaud's phenomenon<br>◆ Rash associated with muscle pain, tenderness, and induration |
| **Postherpetic neuralgia** | |
| Varicella virus in ganglia of posterior nerve roots that reactivates, multiplies, and spreads down sensory nerves to skin. Complication of chronic phase of herpes zoster. | ◆ Intractable neurologic pain (lasts over 6 weeks after disappearance of herpes zoster rash) |
| **Proctitis** | |
| Acute or chronic inflammation of rectal mucosa. Contributing factors that allow normal mucosa to break down include trauma, infection, allergies, drugs, radiation, and sexually transmitted diseases. | ◆ Mild pain, mucus discharge, or bleeding of rectum; feeling of rectal fullness; tenesmus<br>◆ Urge to pass feces with inability to do so<br>◆ Pus, blood, or mucus in stools |

| Pathophysiology | Signs and symptoms |
|---|---|

### *Pseudogout*
Condition in which calcium pyrophosphate crystals deposit in periarticular joint structures, commonly invading knee joint. Associated with conditions that cause degenerative or metabolic changes in cartilage.

◆ Sudden joint pain and swelling in larger peripheral joints (mimics arthritis)

### *Pseudomembranous enterocolitis*
Acute inflammation and necrosis of small and large intestines, usually affecting mucosa. Necrotic mucosa is replaced by pseudomembrane filled with staphylococci, leukocytes, mucus, fibrin, and inflammatory cells. May be caused by toxin produced by *Clostridium difficile.*

◆ Copious watery or bloody diarrhea, abdominal pain, fever
◆ Possible severe dehydration, electrolyte imbalance, hypotension, shock, and colonic perforation

### *Ptosis*
Stretching of eyelid skin or aponeurotic tendon, causing upper eyelid to droop. Lesion affects innervation of either of two muscles that open eyelid. May be congenital or result from mechanical, myogenic, neurogenic, or nutritional factors.

◆ Drooping of upper eyelid

### *Pyloric stenosis*
Obstruction of pyloric orifice of stomach in which pyloric sphincter muscle fibers thicken and become inelastic, leading to narrowed opening. Extra peristaltic effort needed leads to hypertrophied stomach muscle layers.

◆ Progressive nonbilious vomiting, leading to projectile vomiting (at ages 2 to 4 weeks)

### *Rectal prolapse*
Circumferential protrusion of one or more mucous membrane layers through anus due to conditions that increase intra-abdominal pressure within pelvic floor or rectum.

◆ Lower abdominal pain (due to ulceration), bloody diarrhea, tissue protruding from rectum (during defecation or walking)

| Pathophysiology | Signs and symptoms |
|---|---|

### Reiter's syndrome

Infection (caused by *Mycoplasma, Shigella, Salmonella, Yersinia,* or *Chlamydia* organisms) that may initiate aberrant and hyperactive immune response, producing inflammation in involved target organs.

*General symptoms:*
- ◆ Low-grade fever, unexplained diarrhea
- ◆ Superficial lesions on palms or soles

*Genitourinary symptoms:*
- ◆ Burning sensation during urination, penile discharge, and prostatitis (in men)
- ◆ Cervicitis, urethritis, and vulvovaginitis (in women)

*Joint symptoms:*
- ◆ Inflammation where tendon attaches to bone (knees, ankles, feet)

*Eye symptoms:*
- ◆ Conjunctivitis, uveitis

### Renal infarction

Formation of coagulated, necrotic area in one or both kidneys. Results from renal blood vessel occlusion that reduces blood flow to renal tissue and leads to ischemia. Location and size of infarction depend on site of vascular occlusion; usually, infarction affects renal cortex, but it can extend into medulla. Residual renal function after infarction depends on extent of damage from infarction.

- ◆ Severe abdominal or gnawing flank pain and tenderness, costovertebral tenderness
- ◆ Fever, anorexia, nausea, vomiting
- ◆ Possible gross hematuria

### Renal tubular acidosis

Metabolic acidosis resulting from impaired renal function. In type I, distal tubule is unable to secrete hydrogen ions across tubular membrane, causing decreased excretion of titratable acids and ammonium and increased loss of potassium and bicarbonate. Prolonged acidosis leads to hypercalciuria and renal calculi. In type II, defective resorption of bicarbonate in proximal tubule causes bicarbonate to flood distal tubule, leading to impaired formation of titratable acids and ammonium for excretion.

*In infants:*
- ◆ Vomiting, fever, constipation, anorexia, weakness, polyuria, growth retardation, nephrocalcinosis, rickets

*In children and adults:*
- ◆ Growth problems, urinary tract infection, rickets

| **Pathophysiology** | **Signs and symptoms** |
|---|---|

### Renal vein thrombosis

Clotting in renal vein that results in renal congestion, engorgement, and possible infarction. May be acute or chronic, affecting both kidneys. Chronic thrombosis usually impairs renal function, causing nephrotic syndrome. Abrupt onset with extensive damage may precipitate rapidly fatal renal infarction. Less severe thrombosis (affecting only one kidney) or gradual progression (allowing circulation to develop) may preserve partial renal function.

*Rapid onset:*
◆ Severe lumbar pain and tenderness in epigastric region and costovertebral angle
◆ Fever, leukocytosis, pallor, hematuria, proteinuria, peripheral edema
◆ Enlarged kidneys (easily palpable)
*Gradual onset:*
◆ Symptoms of nephrotic syndrome
◆ Pain (possible but generally absent)
◆ Proteinuria, hypoalbuminemia, hyperlipidemia
*In infants:*
◆ Enlarged kidneys, oliguria
◆ Renal insufficiency (may progress to acute or chronic renal failure)

### Renovascular hypertension

Condition marked by rise in systemic blood pressure from stenosis of major renal arteries or their branches or from intrarenal atherosclerosis. Stenosis or occlusion of renal artery stimulates affected kidney to release renin (enzyme that converts angiotensinogen to angiotensin I). As angiotensin I circulates through lungs and liver, it converts to angiotensin II, which causes peripheral vasoconstriction, increased arterial pressure and aldosterone secretion and, eventually, hypertension.

◆ Elevated systemic blood pressure
◆ Headache, palpitations, tachycardia, anxiety, light-headedness, decreased tolerance of temperature extremes, retinopathy, mental sluggishness

### Retinal detachment

Separation of neural retina from underlying retinal pigment epithelium. Caused by trauma (including cataract surgery), severe uveitis, or primary or metastatic choroidal tumors. May also occur from internal changes in vitreous chamber associated with aging.

◆ Floaters, flashing lights
◆ Gradual, painless vision loss (scotoma in peripheral visual field or appearance of "curtain" or "veil" in field of vision)

| **Pathophysiology** | **Signs and symptoms** |
|---|---|

### Retinitis pigmentosa

Inherited disorder in which slow, degenerative changes in rods cause retina and pigment epithelium to atrophy. This produces irregular black deposits of clumped pigment in equatorial region of retina and eventually in macular and peripheral areas.

◆ Progressive night blindness, visual field constriction with ring scotoma, loss of acuity progressing to blindness

### Rocky Mountain spotted fever

Tick-borne disease in which *Rickettsia rickettsii* multiplies within endothelial cells and spreads via bloodstream. Focal areas of infiltration lead to thrombosis and leakage of red blood cells into surrounding tissue.

◆ Fever, headache, mental confusion, myalgia
◆ Rash (appearance of small macules that progress to maculopapules and petechiae, beginning on wrists and ankles and spreading to trunk; diagnostic rash on palms and soles)
◆ Constipation, abdominal distention

### Rosacea

Chronic skin eruption that produces flushing from dilation of small blood vessels in face, especially nose and cheeks. May be aggravated by anything that produces flushing (hot beverages, tobacco, alcohol, spicy foods, physical activity, sunlight, and extreme heat or cold).

◆ Pronounced flushing of nose, cheeks, and forehead
◆ Papules, pustules, telangiectases (may be superimposed)

### Sarcoidosis

Multisystemic, granulomatous disorder that characteristically produces lymphadenopathy, pulmonary infiltration, and skeletal, liver, eye, or skin lesions. Organ dysfunction results from accumulation of T lymphocytes, mononuclear phagocytes, and nonsecreting epithelial granulomas, which distort normal tissue architecture. May result from exaggerated cellular immune response to limited class of antigens.

◆ Respiratory symptoms (generalized, mosty involving lung)
◆ Fever, fatigue, malaise

| **Pathophysiology** | **Signs and symptoms** |
|---|---|

### Scabies

Highly transmissible skin infestation of *Sarcoptes scabiei* in which mites burrow superficially beneath stratum corneum, depositing eggs that hatch, mature, and reinvade skin. Sensitization reaction against mite excreta results.

◆ Intense itching (worsens at night)
◆ Threadlike lesions (on wrists, between fingers, and on elbows, axillae, belt line, buttocks, and male genitalia)
◆ Possible secondary bacterial infection

### Schistosomiasis

Parasitic infestation of blood flukes usually due to bathing with free-swimming larvae (cercariae) of Trematoda class, which penetrate skin, migrate to intrahepatic portal circulation, and mature. Adult worms lodge in venules of bladder or intestines.

*Initial stage:*
◆ Pruritic papular dermatitis (at penetration site), fever, cough
*Later stage:*
◆ Hepatosplenomegaly, lymphadenopathy
◆ Possible seizures and skin abscesses

### Scleroderma

Diffuse connective tissue disease characterized by fibrotic, degenerative, and occasionally inflammatory changes in skin, blood vessels, synovial membranes, skeletal muscles, and internal organs (especially esophagus, intestinal tract, thyroid, heart, lungs, and kidneys).

◆ Raynaud's phenomenon, progressive phalangeal resorption (may shorten fingers)
◆ Slow healing of ulcers on fingertips or toes (may lead to gangrene due to poor circulation)
◆ Pain, stiffness, and swelling of fingers and joints (occurs later)
◆ Skin thickening (produces taut, shiny skin over entire hand and forearm); facial skin disfigurement (becomes tight and inelastic, causing masklike appearance and "pinching" of mouth)
◆ GI dysfunction: frequent reflux, heartburn, dysphagia, and bloating after meals
◆ Arrhythmias and dyspnea (with advanced disease)

| Pathophysiology | Signs and symptoms |
|---|---|

### Septic arthritis

Infectious disorder in which bacteria (gram-positive cocci, *Staphylococcus aureus, Streptococcus pyogenes* and *pneumoniae* in children; *Neisseria gonor-rhoeae, S. aureus,* and sptreptococci in adults) invade joint, causing inflammation of synovial lining, effusion and pyogene-sis, and destruction of bone and cartilage. Medical emergency that can lead to anky-losis, even fatal septicemia, without prompt treatment.

◆ Intense pain, inflammation, and swelling of affected joint
◆ Low-grade fever
◆ Migratory polyarthritis

### Severe combined immunodeficiency syndrome

Deficiency or absence of cell-mediated (T-cell) and humoral (B-cell) immunity that predisposes patient to infection from all classes of microorganisms during infancy. In most cases, genetic defect seems associated with failure of stem cell to differentiate into T and B lymphocytes. Many molecular defects, such as mutation of the kinase ZAP-70, can cause this disor-der. X-linked severe combined immuno-deficiency syndrome is due to mutation of a subunit of interleukin (IL)-2, IL-4, and IL-7 receptors. Less commonly, it results from an enzyme deficiency.

◆ Extreme susceptibility to infection
◆ Failure to thrive and chronic otitis, sep-sis, and watery diarrhea (associated with *Salmonella* or *Escherichia coli*); recurrent pulmonary infections, persis-tent oral candidiasis, and potentially fatal viral infections (chickenpox)
◆ *Pneumocystis carinii* pneumonia

### Shigellosis

Acute infectious inflammatory colitis caused by oral ingestion or transmission via fecal-oral route of *Shigella* organisms. Causes high fever (especially in children) and acute, self-limiting diarrhea and tenesmus; may also cause electrolyte imbalance and dehydration. Invasion of colonic epithelial cells and cell-to-cell spread of infection results in characteristic mucosal ulcerations.

*In children:*
◆ Fever, watery diarrhea, nausea, vomit-ing, irritability, abdominal pain and dis-tention
*In adults:*
◆ Intermittent severe abdominal pain, tenesmus and (in severe cases) headache and prostration; fever (rare)
◆ Pus, blood, or mucus in stools

| Pathophysiology | Signs and symptoms |
|---|---|

### Silicosis
Progressive disease (most common form of pneumoconiosis) caused by exposure to silica dust and characterized by nodular lesions that frequently lead to fibrosis. Alveolar macrophages engulf respirable particles of free silica, causing release of cytotoxic enzymes. This attracts other macrophages and produces fibrous tissue in lung parenchyma. Associated with high incidence of active tuberculosis.

*In simple nodular silicosis:*
◆ Cough, sputum
*In conglomerate silicosis:*
◆ Severe shortness of breath and cough, excessive sputum (may lead to pulmonary hypertension and cor pulmonale)

### Sjögren's syndrome
Autoimmune rheumatic disorder characterized by lymphocytic infiltration of exocrine glands, causing tissue damage resulting in xerostomia and dry eyes.

*In xerostomia:*
◆ Dry mouth; difficulty swallowing and speaking; ulcers of tongue, buccal mucosa, and lips; severe dental caries
*In ocular involvement:*
◆ Eye dryness, sensation of grit or sand in eyes
◆ Decreased tearing; burning, itching, or redness; photosensitivity
*Extraglandular:*
◆ Arthralgia, Raynaud's phenomenon, lymphadenopathy, lung involvement

### Sleep apnea
Cessation of airflow during sleep caused by upper airway narrowing or glottal obstruction as result of obesity or congenital abnormalities of upper airway. When primary brain stem medullary failure occurs, sleeping patient may breathe insufficiently or not at all.

*In obstructive sleep apnea:*
◆ Snoring, excessive daytime sleepiness, intellectual impairment, memory loss, cardiopulmonary symptoms
*In central sleep apnea:*
◆ Sleep disturbances, morning headache, daytime fatigue

### Spinal ischemia
Condition in which major arterial branches that supply spinal cord become compressed or occluded, decreasing blood flow to spinal cord, causing cord ischemia and motor and sensory deficiencies. Caused by vascular compression (tumors and acute disc compression) or by remote occlusion (aortic surgery and dissecting aneurysm).

◆ Sudden back pain, pain around affected segment
◆ Bilateral flaccid weakness and dissociated sensory loss (below level of infarct)

| Pathophysiology | Signs and symptoms |
| --- | --- |

### Sporotrichosis

Chronic fungal infection caused by inoculation of *Sporothrix schenckii* into subcutaneous tissue through minor trauma. Produces inflammatory response that includes clustering of neutrophils and marked granulomatous response, in which epithelioid cells and giant cells produce nodular erythematous primary lesions and secondary lesions along lymphatic channels (in cutaneous lymphatic type). In pulmonary sporotrichosis, inflammatory response produces pulmonary lesions and nodules. In disseminated sporotrichosis, multifocal lesions spread from skin or lungs.

*In cutaneous or lymphatic sporotrichosis:*
◆ Subcutaneous, movable, painless nodule on hands or fingers (grows progressively larger, discolors, and eventually ulcerates); additional lesions (on adjacent lymph node chain)
*In pulmonary sporotrichosis:*
◆ Productive cough, pleural effusion, fibrosis, formation of fungus ball
*In disseminated sporotrichosis:*
◆ Weight loss, anorexia, synovial or bony lesions, possible arthritis or osteomyelitis

### Stickler syndrome

Inherited chondrodysplasia caused by structural defects in collagen, an essential component of connective tissue. Characterized by ocular, skeletal, auditory, and cranial abnormalities. Collagen defect typically is caused by mutation in type II collagen gene (COL2A1) located on chromosome 12q13.11 to 12q13.2. Others show linkage to the COL11A2 gene located on chromosome 6p21.3 and others to COL11A1 gene located on chromosome 1p21. COL11A2 and COL11A1 are expressed in the hyaline cartilage, vitreous, intervertebral disc, and inner ear.

◆ Ocular symptoms: myopia, vitreal abnormalities, and retinal detachment resulting in blindness
◆ Auditory symptoms: conductive hearing loss or sensorineural hearing loss
◆ Craniofacial features: micrognathia (unusually small jaw), flattened midface and nasal bridge
◆ Skeletal symptoms: joint hypermobility, spondyloepiphyseal dysplasia, degenerative arthropathy

### Stomatitis

Inflammation of cells of oral mucosa, buccal mucosa, lips, and palate that results in ulcer formation. Caused by herpes simplex virus.

◆ Papulovesicular ulcers (in mouth and throat), mouth pain, malaise, anorexia, swelling of mucous membranes

| **Pathophysiology** | **Signs and symptoms** |
|---|---|

### Strabismus

Commonly inherited disorder characterized by malalignment of eye. In paralytic (nonconcomitant) strabismus, paralysis of one or more ocular muscles may be due to oculomotor nerve lesion. In nonparalytic (concomitant) strabismus, unequal ocular muscle tone is due to supranuclear abnormality within CNS.

◆ Eye malalignment (noticeable upon external eye examination), corneal light reflex in center of pupils (upon ophthalmoscopic examination), diplopia, visual disturbances
◆ Diminished visual acuity (with decreased use of one eye)

### Thrombocythemia

Clonal abnormality of multipotent hematopoietic stem cells that results in increased platelet production, although platelet survival is usually normal. If combined with degenerative vascular disease, may lead to serious bleeding or thrombosis.

◆ Weakness, hemorrhage, nonspecific headache, paresthesia, dizziness, easy bruising

### Thrombophlebitis

Inflammation of vein associated with thrombus formation. Alteration in epithelial lining causes platelet aggregation and fibrin entrapment of red and white blood cells and additional platelets; thrombus initiates chemical inflammatory process in vessel's epithelium that leads to fibrosis, which may occlude vessel lumen or embolize.

◆ Extreme tenderness, swelling, and redness at affected site

### Tinea versicolor

Nondermatophyte dimorphic fungus that converts to hyphal form and causes characteristic lesions. Invasion of stratum corneum by yeast produces C9and C11 dicarboxylic acids that inhibit tyrosinase in vitro.

◆ Well-delineated, hyperpigmented or hypopigmented macules (on upper trunk and arms)

| Pathophysiology | Signs and symptoms |
|---|---|

### *Torticollis*

Contraction of sternocleidomastoid neck muscles that produces twisting of neck and unnatural head position. May be congenital (prenatal malposition or injury, fibroma, interrupted blood supply) or acquired (inflammatory disease or cervical spinal lesions that produce scar tissue).

*Congenital:*
◆ Firm, nontender, palpable enlargement of sternocleidomastoid muscle (visible at birth)
*Acquired:*
◆ Recurrent unilateral stiffness of neck muscles
◆ "Drawing" sensation (pulling of head to affected side)
◆ Severe neuralgic pain of head and neck

### *Tourette syndrome*

Inherited chronic disorder that produces characteristic motor and phonic tics. Obscure pathology; however, dopaminergic excess may be a factor (tics may respond to treatment with dopamine-blocking drugs).

◆ Single or multiple motor tics (commonly affect face), phonic tics
◆ Involuntary arm and shoulder movements

### *Trachoma*

Chronic conjunctivitis due to *Chlamydia trachomatis* that leads to inflammatory leukocytic infiltration and superficial vascularization of cornea, conjunctival scarring, and eyelid distortion. Causes lashes to abrade cornea, which progresses to corneal ulceration, scarring, and blindness.

◆ Mild infection resembling bacterial conjunctivitis; red and edematous eyelids; eye pain, tearing, and exudation; photophobia

### *Trichomoniasis*

Infection of genitourinary tract (vagina, urethra and, possibly, endocervix, bladder, or Bartholin's or Skene's glands) due to *Trichomonas vaginalis*. In males, causes infection of lower urethra and possibly prostate gland, seminal vesicles, and epididymis.

*In females:*
◆ Malodorous, greenish-yellow vaginal discharge; irritation of vulva, perineum, and thighs; dyspareunia; dysuria
*In males:*
◆ Generally asymptomatic; possible transient frothy or purulent urethral discharge with dysuria and frequency; recurrent urethritis

| Pathophysiology | Signs and symptoms |
|---|---|

### *Trigeminal neuralgia*

Painful disorder along distribution of one or more of trigeminal nerve's sensory divisions (usually maxillary). May result from compression neuropathy.

◆ Searing or burning pain (lasts seconds to 2 minutes at trigeminal nerve distribution)
◆ Painful response (upon touching trigger point)

### *Uterine leiomyomas*

Benign tumors of smooth muscle of uterus (submucosal, intramural, subserosal); also found in broad ligaments and, rarely, in cervix. Linked to steroid hormones and growth factors.

◆ Abnormal bleeding (common)
◆ Pain or pressure at tumor site
◆ Urinary or bowel disturbances

### *Uveitis*

Inflammation of any part of uveal tract. Inflammatory cells floating in aqueous humor or deposited on corneal endothelium affect uveal tract. Associated with autoimmune diseases, allergies, infections, chemicals, trauma, and surgery.

*Anterior:*
◆ Eye pain or redness, photophobia, and decreased vision
*Intermediate:*
◆ Floaters and decreased vision
*Posterior:*
◆ Floaters and decreased vision (most common; other diverse symptoms possible)

### *Vaginal cancer*

Tumor development in vagina that presents mainly as squamous cell carcinoma (sometimes as melanoma, sarcoma, or adenocarcinoma) and progresses from intraepithelial tumor to invasive cancer.

◆ Abnormal bleeding and discharge
◆ Firm, ulcerated lesion in vagina

### *Vaginismus*

Involuntary spastic constriction of lower vaginal muscles, tightly closing vaginal introitus.

◆ Muscle spasm with pain (upon vaginal insertion)
◆ Lack of sexual interest or desire

### *Variola*

Viral infection due to variola poxvirus that is transmitted by respiratory droplets or direct contact. Replicates in body and causes viremia.

◆ Fever, vomiting, sore throat, CNS symptoms (headache, malaise, stupor, and coma), macular rash (progresses to vesicular rash), pustular lesions

| Pathophysiology | Signs and symptoms |
|---|---|

### Velocardiofacial syndrome

Chromosomal microdeletion syndrome caused by deletion of chromosome 22q1 1.2. Deletion is submicroscopic (too small to be detected by routine chromosome analysis); deleted region, containing 1.5 to 3 megabases, is thought to contain a number of genes. Because infants with DiGeorge syndrome often test positive for a 22q1 1.2 deletion, DiGeorge syndrome represents severe end of syndrome's clinical spectrum.

◆ Severe form: complex heart malformations, dysmorphic features, hypocalcemia, missing thymus, renal abnormalities
◆ Cardiac anomalies: conotruncal defects (tetralogy of Fallot, interrupted aortic arch, truncus arteriosus)
◆ Craniofacial features: abnormal palate, dysmorphic facial features, dysphagia
◆ Neuropsychological symptoms: hypotonia, cognitive symptoms, psychiatric disorders

### Vitiligo

Destruction of melanocytes (humoral or cellular) and circulating antibodies against melanocytes that results in hypopigmented areas.

◆ Progressive areas of complete pigment loss (usually symmetrical, with sharp borders; generally appear in periorificial areas, flexor wrists, and extensor distal extremities)

### Volvulus

Twisting of intestinal tract at least 180 degrees on its mesentery, causing blood vessel compression and ischemia. In adults, most common site is sigmoid bowel; in children, small bowel. Other common sites include stomach and cecum.

◆ Vomiting
◆ Rapid, marked abdominal distention; sudden, severe abdominal pain

### Vulval cancer

Slow-growing squamous or basal cell cancer that usually begins on skin surface and, untreated, spreads to vagina, urethra, anus, or lymph nodes.

◆ Unusual lumps or sores
◆ Vulvar pruritus
◆ Bleeding
◆ Small painful, infected ulcer
◆ Groin pain
◆ Abnormal urination and defecation

### Vulvovaginitis

Inflammation of vulva and vaginal mucosa resulting from bacterial or viral infection, vaginal atrophy, or various traumas or irritations.

◆ Vaginal discharge (consistency, odor, and color vary with causative agent)
◆ Possible vulvar irritation, pain, or pruritus

| **Pathophysiology** | **Signs and symptoms** |
|---|---|

### Wilson's disease

Excessive copper retention in liver, kidneys, brain, and cornea resulting from defective mobilization of copper from hepatocellular lysosomes for excretion via bile. Causes tissue necrosis and subsequent hepatic and neurologic disorders.

◆ Kayser-Fleischer ring (rusty-brown pigmented ring at periphery of corneas)
◆ Signs of hepatitis leading to cirrhosis
◆ Tremors, unsteady gait, muscle rigidity
◆ Inappropriate behavior, psychosis
◆ Hematuria, proteinuria, uricosuria

### Wiskott-Aldrich syndrome

X-linked recessive immunodeficiency disorder characterized by defective B- and T-cell function and susceptibility to infection. Metabolic defect in platelet synthesis causes production of small, short-lived platelets, resulting in thrombocytopenia.

*In neonates:*
◆ Hemorrhagic symptoms (bloody stools, bleeding from circumcision site, petechiae, and purpura)
*In older children:*
◆ Recurrent systemic infections, eczema

### X-linked infantile hypogammaglobulinemia

Congenital disorder characterized by deficiency or absence of B cells, leading to defective immune response and depressed production of all five immunoglobulin types.

◆ Recurrent infections (beginning at about age 6 months): otitis media, pneumonia, dermatitis, bronchitis, meningitis, conjunctivitis, abnormal dental caries, polyarthritis

# Selected references

*Atlas of Pathophysiology,* 2nd ed. Philadelphia: Lippincott Williams & Wilkins, 2005.

Becker, K.L., et al. *Principles and Practice of Endocrinology and Metabolism,* 3rd ed. Philadelphia: Lippincott Williams & Wilkins, 2003.

Beutler, E., et al., eds. *Williams' Hematology,* 6th ed. New York: McGraw-Hill Book Co., 2001.

Braunwald, E., et al., eds. *Harrison's Principles of Internal Medicine,* 15th ed. New York: McGraw-Hill Book Co., 2001.

Brunwald, E., et al., eds. *Heart Disease: A Textbook of Cardiovascular Medicine,* 6th ed. Philadelphia: W.B. Saunders Co., 2001.

*Critical Care Challenges: Disorders, Treatments, and Procedures.* Philadelphia: Lippincott Williams & Wilkins, 2003.

*Critical Care Nursing Made Incredibly Easy!* Philadelphia: Lippincott Williams & Wilkins, 2003.

*Fluids and Electrolytes Made Incredibly Easy!,* 2nd ed. Springhouse, Pa: Springhouse Corp., 2002.

Gould, B.E. *Pathophysiology for Health Care Professionals,* 2nd ed. Philadelphia: W.B. Saunders Co., 2002.

Ignatavicius, D.D., and Workman, M.L. *Medical-Surgical Nursing: Critical Thinking for Collaborative Care,* 4th ed. Philadelphia: W.B. Saunders Co., 2002.

Johnson, R.J., and Feehally, J., eds. *Comprehensive Clinical Nephrology,* 2nd ed. St. Louis: Mosby-Year Book, Inc., 2003.

*Nursing2005 Drug Handbook.* Philadelphia: Lippincott Williams & Wilkins, 2005.

Patton, S.E., et al. "Bladder Cancer," *Current Opinion in Oncology* 14(3): 265-72, May 2002.

Paul, W.E. *Fundamental Immunology,* 5th ed. Philadelphia: Lippincott Williams & Wilkins, 2003.

*Physicians Desk Reference 2004, 58th ed.* Montvale, N.J.: Thomson PDR, 2004.

Porth, C.M. *Essentials of Pathophysiology: Concepts of Altered Health States,* 6th ed. Philadelphia: Lippincott Williams & Wilkins, 2002.

*Professional Guide to Pathophysiology.* Philadelphia: Lippincott Williams & Wilkins, 2003.

Skidmore-Roth, L. *2003 Mosby Nursing Drug Reference.* St. Louis: Mosby-Year Book, Inc., 2002.

Smith, G. *Gastrointestinal Nursing.* Cambridge, Mass.: Blackwell Scientific Pubns., 2004.

Tierney, L.M., et al., eds. *Current Medical Diagnosis and Treatment 2003.* Stamford, Conn.: Appleton & Lange, 2003.

Ware, L.B., and Matthay, M.A. "The Acute Respiratory Distress Syndrome," *New England Journal of Medicine* 342(18):1334-49, May 4, 2000.

Yamada, T., et al. *Textbook of Gastroenterology,* 4th ed. Philadelphia: Lippincott Williams & Wilkins, 2003.

Zychowicz, M.E., ed. *Orthopedic Nursing Secrets.* Philadelphia: Elsevier Science, 2003.

# ᴬdex

## A

Abdominal aortic aneurysm, 9-10, 9i
Acetylcholine, in myasthenia gravis, 109i
Acid-base disorders, 311-361
   pathophysiologic concepts of, 312-313
Acidosis, 312
   metabolic, 346-349, 346i-347i
   respiratory, 354-358, 354i-356i
Acquired immunodeficiency syndrome, 192-194, 192i
Acute coronary syndrome, 6-8, 6i
Acute lymphocytic leukemia, 179
Acute myelogenous leukemia, 179
Acute poststreptococcal glomerulonephritis, 245
Acute renal failure, 232-235, 232i
Acute respiratory distress syndrome, 51-53, 51i
Acute tubular necrosis, 236-238, 236i
Acute tubulointerstitial nephritis, 236
Addison's disease, 210
Addisonian crisis, 210
Adenoid hyperplasia, 364
Adrenal crisis, 210, 211i, 212
Adrenal hypofunction, 210-213, 211i
Adrenogenital syndrome, 364
Agnosia, 89
Albinism, 364
Alkalosis, 312
   metabolic, 350-353, 350i-351i
   respiratory, 359-361, 359i-360i
Alpha₁-antitrypsin deficiency, 364
Alveolus, 72i
Alzheimer's disease, 90-92, 90i
Amblyopia, 365
Amyloidosis, 365
Amyloid plaques, 90i
Amyotrophic lateral sclerosis, 93-94, 93i

Anaphylaxis, 195-198, 195i-196i
Anasarca, 312
Anemia, 165
   folic acid deficiency, 166-167, 166i
   iron deficiency, 168-170, 168i
   pernicious, 171-173, 171i
   sickle cell, 308-310, 308i
Anencephaly, 305, 306
Aneurysm, 2-3, 2i
   abdominal aortic, 9-10, 9i
   intracranial, 95-97, 95i
Angina, 7
   management of, 8
Ankylosing spondylitis, 365
Anorexia, 121
Antidiuretic hormone secretion, excessive, 226
Aortic aneurysm
   abdominal, 9-10, 9i
   types of, 2i
Aortic insufficiency, 11-13, 11i
Aortic stenosis, 14-15, 14i
Aphasia, 89
Apnea, sleep, 391
Arousal, altered, 86
Arterial pressure, mean, 230
Artery, pulmonary, 78i
Arthritis
   rheumatoid, 199-201, 199i
   septic, 390
Aspergillosis, 366
Asthma, 54-56, 54i
Atelectasis, 49
Atrophy, 249
   muscle, 149
Aura, in migraine headache, 103
Autoimmune reactions, 190
Autosomal disorders, 290

## B

Bacterial pneumonia, 66i
Basal cell carcinoma, 250-252, 250i
B-cell hyperactivity, 190

---

i refers to an illustration; t refers to a table.

i refers to an illustration; t refers to a table.

i refers to an illustration; t refers to a table.

---

i refers to an illustration; t refers to a table.

i refers to an illustration; t refers to a table.

i refers to an illustration; t refers to a table.

i refers to an illustration; t refers to a table.